BODYCRAFT

Health and Beauty the Natural Way

BODYCRAFT

Health and Beauty the Natural Way

NERYS PURCHON

PHOTOGRAPHY BY QUENTIN BACON

STYLING BY LOUISE OWENS

ILLUSTRATIONS BY
DIANNE BRADLEY AND JANET JONES

Blitz Editions

ACKNOWLEDGEMENTS

My love and thanks to Prakash, who has once again lived, supported and suffered through another manuscript! To Nirala for her ever ready and efficient help and friendship, and to Amber who became a 'sorcerer's apprentice'.

Thanks once again to Fred Kraeter—you never let me down; to Carol Turner who read my chapter on food and diet and who offered practical and intelligent suggestions, and to Dr Bruce Sunderland of Curtin University who, patiently and in terms which I could understand, answered my questions on chemistry. Thanks to Joe Patroni of the WA Department of Agriculture for his information regarding lanolin, and to Steve Noblett of Spectrum.

Finally to a dozen or more people to whom I turned for information on subjects as diverse as margarine and preservatives, and who gave unstintingly of their knowledge and advice—I thank you all.

Editor: Jan Castorina
Designers: Liz Seymour, Anna Soo
Assistant Designer: Raylee Sloane
Editorial Assistant: Ella Martin
Stylist's Assistants: Dimity Green, Amanda Greenfield

Published By Blitz Editions
an imprint of
Bookmart Limited
Registered Number 2372865
Trading as Bookmart Limited
Desford Road
Enderby
Leicester
LE9 5AD

First published in 1993 by Hodder & Stoughton (Aust.) Pty Ltd.
This edition published in Australia in 1995
by Hodder Headline Australia Pty Limited
10–16 South Street, Rydalmere, NSW, 2116.

ISBN 1 85605 327 X

Printed in Hong Kong
Produced in Hong Kong by Mandarin Offset

PREFACE

Some of the happiest years of my life were spent on a small farm called Rivendell where Prakash (my husband) and I, together with family and friends, had a small cosmetic company making natural, herbal and cruelty-free products.

At the farm we also ran a restaurant called The Prancing Pony where we served meals which specialised in fruit, vegetables and herbs from our gardens and orchard.

There could have been few less likely places to run a business or a restaurant but because we were totally involved in, and in love with, what we were doing, it worked, and worked well. The contents of this book are largely the result of the many things I learnt during this special and fulfulling time.

I now live in a motor home travelling the roads of Australia. I run aromatherapy and herbcraft courses wherever I can and continue to make many preparations for cooking, healing, cleaning, deodorising and sweetening the air, bathing, hair care, skin care, perfuming linen and stationery, and deterring insects from eating us, our books and clothes!

I wrote my first book, Herbcraft, in order to share with you my love, enthusiasm and respect for herbs. Foodcraft, my second book, was about another love of mine: cooking, eating and sharing food and drink with my family and friends — herbs were strongly featured in this second book also. Aromatherapy was conceived many years ago during walks through scented gardens and forests and eventuated in 1994.

Bodycraft embraces all of the above and more. Upon making the preparations in this book, Mother Nature hands over and you become the Sorcerer, turning the herbs and other plants, oils and essences into those magical things which will save your money, cherish your body, soothe your mind and put you in touch with your spirit.

This book is dedicated to Eeyore, Pooh, Tigger and Piglet, the first members of the
'House at Pooh Corner', and to Roo who joined the family at a later date and enriched
it beyond measure. I love you and thank you for choosing me—without you my life
would have been meaningless.

CONTENTS

CONTENTS

Flowers by Lisa Milasas

INTRODUCTION

First we will start with beauty's care,
For beauty is the grace of heaven;
Well-tended vines productive are,
To well-tilled fields good crops are given;
And so with beauty: but how few
Can show a cheek of perfect hue!
—OVID (43BC–?17AD)

Down the centuries the poets have eulogised beauty, minstrels have sung of it, artists have tried to capture it on canvas and billions of dollars are spent each year all over the world by men and women in the search for beautiful skin and thick glossy hair. The production and making of skin and hair preparations is a very big business.

In this search, we often confuse beauty with youth, as this is the time when we remember our lips being rosy, cheeks glowing, skin fresh, firm and dewy, and hair a thick mane of curls and waves or a fall of shining silk. Eyes were bright and clear and bodies firm and strong. We conveniently forget the teenage spots, insecurity and 'puberty blues'. What we are yearning for is the appearance of youth which comes from glowing health.

It can be very demoralising if we waste our time trying to 'turn back the clock', but if we take good care of our bodies, minds and souls in the most natural way possible we will gain satisfaction and added self-esteem in our improved appearance, health and contentment, and in the knowledge that we are in control of our lives.

We may have a specific reason to begin a programme of self-improvement: puffing when we walk fast; no longer fitting into last year's clothes; an awareness that we are eating unsuitable food and often too much of it; skin looking jaded, lifeless or spotty; worrying continually; we can't sleep, and spend our days in a daze of exhaustion; we're sick of paying exorbitant prices for skin- and hair-care products which promise us the earth and don't deliver.

The person we can create is one who exercises regularly for fun and enjoys the feeling of well-being that exercise gives; eats delicious food which is easy to prepare and doesn't clog arteries and put 'saddle bags' on bottoms; is wearing the same size clothes as they wore when they were twenty years old; puts worries in perspective and is learning how to deal with them; sleeps soundly until they want to wake; makes their own skin- and hair-care products which are superior to the bought variety and save money; is proud to be the person they are, the age they are and smiles a lot!

The making of all the preparations in this book can take place at the kitchen stove and sink. The recipes are generally no more difficult than cooking a meal and are often much simpler.

A word of warning: if you are using the kitchen to make your products, do caution family and friends not to taste anything. A friend came to visit, I was on the phone and called to her to put the kettle on. I was alarmed to hear spitting, gargling and choking sounds coming from the kitchen. I raced to the rescue to find that this inquisitive friend had surreptitiously swallowed a big spoonful of the delicious-looking tomato soup on the stove. Problem was that the soup was red candle mix!

Some ingredients, terms and methods might be unfamiliar at first. You would be wise to consult the Glossary for further information.

Jars from The Bay Tree; scent sachets, soap dish and timber bathmat from Lace of Balmain; flowers by Lisa Milasas

CHAPTER ONE

MAKING LOTIONS AND POTIONS

You will feel enriched beyond measure when you, your home and your family and friends are using the gifts of the earth to improve your lives. It is a very special experience to see the raw materials transformed into beautiful and richly scented unguents, perfumes, sachets, room fresheners and other lovely things. The big bonus is that it's not difficult and it's not expensive. This chapter shows how to make the basics needed for making your own products.

Jars from The Bay Tree; flowers by Lisa Milasas

A selection of the basics used in making lotions and potions

EQUIPMENT

I have a special cupboard in which I store all my ingredients and equipment. It's wise to keep special equipment for making the recipes as the powerfully perfumed essential oils are absorbed into wooden utensils and will ruin food with their strong perfumes. Beeswax is very difficult to clean off pans and dishes so it's best to save those pans for recipes containing beeswax.

Search the secondhand shops or buy new:

1–2 funnels	Rubber spatulas
Scissors	Sharp knives
2–3 measuring jugs	2–3 mixing bowls
Tea towels	Crock-pot
Scales	Set of measuring cups
Coffee filter papers	Labels for jars

Big and little pans (not aluminium)
Wooden spoons, teaspoons, tablespoons
Sieves—coarse, medium and fine
Mortar and pestle or electric coffee grinder
Screw-top jars and bottles—different sizes
Amber and dark glass—different sizes
Double boiler (not aluminium)
Deep baking dish or electric frypan
Preserving/jam making or laboratory
    thermometer (two if possible)
Plastic measure (25ml/about 1fl oz)
Eye droppers
Cheesecloth for bags and for fine straining
Waterproof marking pen—fine tip
Electric blender or food processor or whisk

When making preparations which need long, slow and gentle extraction a crock-pot is the perfect utensil. A crock-pot is a large ceramic pot with a lid, which fits into a metal jacket. Under the metal jacket is a thermostatically controlled heating element. Base oils and decoctions are two examples of preparations which can be made in a crock-pot.

You will need a double boiler for some recipes. To hold bowls or jars, an electric frypan half full of water is an ideal arrangement as it frees you from the stove and you could use the laundry.

A deep baking dish half-filled with water and used on the stove is another alternative. If you are making an emulsion you will need two bowls or jars side by side in the water bath The phases will then reach the same temperature.

If you are using a single phase method, a bowl which fits snugly into a pan of water will suffice. Very small amounts may be made in the storage jar by standing it in water in a small shallow pan.

Make sure that all equipment is scrupulously clean before beginning (the saucepans you use for beeswax may have stubborn residue left on them). The cleaner your equipment and jars, the longer your cosmetics will keep fresh.

All glass containers should be washed in soapy water, rinsed, and dried at the bottom of an oven which is set on low. Alternatively, the bottles or jars can be boiled in water for 20 minutes (place on a folded cloth in the bottom of the pan). Plastics may be sterilised by soaking in water and sodium metabisulphite (from pharmacies).

STRAINING AND FILTERING

To ensure the longest possible life for preparations, the infusions and oils should be thoroughly strained to remove of any plant matter. With bulk plant material, the quickest method is to strain through two or three different grades of sieve from coarse to fine, and then finally through a coffee filter paper.

Cheesecloth bags are useful if you want to drip and/or strain liquids from materials. Bags are easy to handle; the top can be tied so the ingredients in the bag will not fall into the strained liquid.

The cheesecloth you will need is not the type used to make clothing, but a much cheaper type sometimes known as 'muslin' or 'butter muslin'. To make cheesecloth bags, use double thickness material and French seams. It's a good idea to make several sizes, varying in size from 8cm x 12cm (3in x 5in) up to 18cm x 25cm (7in x 10in).

Some of the equipment needed

HERBS

Gather your herbs from the wild or from the garden. Ensure they are not contaminated by herbicides, pesticides or petrol fumes.

It is important to use the correct part of the plant where the greatest concentration of the active ingredient is to be found. (I have indicated this in the entries on each herb in the Glossary.)

The time of collection is important. Plants are highly active and dynamic—all through the day and night the character and constituents of the plants are changing. These changes also happen from season to season and plants can produce different chemicals at different times of the year. These differences are very important when a plant is being used internally and medicinally, but for the external uses the following is a good guide:

Collect all plant material in the morning when the dew has dried but before the sun is hot.

LEAVES	before flowering. The exceptions are marjoram and oregano; both flowers and leaves may be used.
FLOWERS	when the flower is just fully open.
ROOTS	before the plant flowers.
SEEDS	when fully ripe but before they fall.
BARK	any time as a rule.

Dry the plants in a shady, well-ventilated spot protected from flies and insects. (Check the plants for insects before putting to dry or you might end up providing the bugs with a restaurant.)

Store in glass jars in a cool dark place. Label at every stage from drying to storing.

WEIGHTS AND MEASURES

All spoon and cup measures in this book are standard except where teacups are used. Teacups are used in some recipes to make measuring the ingredients simple, in these cases it does not affect the recipe if the ingredients are a few grams under or over.

A standard cup measure set usually consists of 1 cup, $\frac{1}{2}$ cup, $\frac{1}{3}$ cup and $\frac{1}{4}$ cup. Spoon sets usually contain 1 tablespoon, 1 teaspoon, $\frac{1}{2}$ teaspoon, $\frac{1}{4}$ teaspoon.

CUP SIZES		SPOON SIZES	
Cup	ml	Spoon	ml
$\frac{1}{4}$	60	$\frac{1}{4}$ teaspoon	1.25
$\frac{1}{3}$	80	$\frac{1}{2}$ teaspoon	2.5
$\frac{1}{2}$	125	1 teaspoon	5
1	250	1 tablespoon	20

The following measures will help you when you are mixing and blending essential oils:

18 to 20 drops = 1ml = 1 marked dropper

90 to 100 drops = 5ml = 1 metric teaspoon

20ml = 1 metric tablespoon

A dropper is marked in amounts up to 1ml.

Blue and white saucer from Crabtree & Evelyn; flowers by Lisa Milasas

Various ingredients often used for making lotions and potions

PREPARING BEESWAX

Beeswax can be bought from the pharmacy (expensive) or from a beekeeper (much cheaper). Beeswax from a beekeeper is likely to be full of strange bits and pieces such as bees legs and wings, and flower scraps, and will need thorough cleansing before use.

CLEANSING BEESWAX

Put the beeswax in a large old pan, cover with water and heat very slowly until the wax has melted. Allow to cool. Lift the wax off the surface of the water and scrape away the layer of dark material which will have formed underneath. If you want to, you can repeat this process.

BEESWAX AND COCOA BUTTER CUBES

The reason for making beeswax and cocoa butter cubes is to create manageable amounts of wax, as it is very difficult to cut small pieces from a large block. In many books, recipes demand a tablespoon or teaspoon of grated beeswax or cocoa butter; if you've ever tried to grate either of them you'll discover how inaccurate this method is, as there is rarely any suggestion as to whether the wax should be finely or coarsely grated, loosely or tightly packed.

The method below ensures that a large number of cubes of the same weight can be made in one session. Any other hard substance (such as emulsifying wax) may be treated in this way, making the process much quicker when you want to make a batch of cream or ointment.

Melt the cleansed wax (very gently or it might burn) and pour it into greased ice cube freezer trays to set. Weigh the resulting cubes (usually about 10–15g ($\frac{1}{3}$–$\frac{1}{2}$oz) each depending on the size of the compartments). Store in an airtight and insect proof container. Write the weight of an average cube on the outside of the container.

PREPARING ALOE

When we owned the cosmetic business Rivendell Farm Skin and Hair Products, we would process huge amount of aloe leaf, chopping the leaves, blending them and straining the pulp. I developed an allergy to the raw pulp. We accidentally found that the finished aloe cream would cure the itching and rash!

The conclusion we reached was that the heating of the pulp in the making of the product destroyed the principle which was responsible for the allergic reaction. In addition to this discovery we noticed that there is a yellow juice held just underneath the skin on the leaf. This yellow juice is incredibly bitter and is—I suspect—responsible for the itching and rash; so if you want to avoid a possible reaction I would suggest that you peel the skin away from the leaf and carefully scrape the jelly centre away, avoiding the yellow juice.

TO PREPARE ALOE FOR USE IN CREAMS AND LOTIONS

Scrape the jelly from the inside of the leaves. Blend the jelly with very little purified water until no lumps remain. Place in a small saucepan and slowly bring to just below boiling point. Allow to go cold. Strain. Refrigerate. Use within 24 hours.

PREPARING FLAX SEEDS

These emollient seeds can be used to make a hair-setting jelly or a soothing skin treatment.

Flax Jelly

Mix $\frac{1}{2}$ cup (90g/3oz) crushed flax seeds with $1\frac{1}{2}$ cups (375ml/12fl oz) water or herb tea. Simmer until it becomes a jelly. Strain and use, or dilute to the desired thickness.

Clockwise from top left: flax seeds, aloe leaves, beeswax cubes and buttons, aloe juice

MAKING EMULSIONS

An emulsion is a mixture of oil and water which, when combined, doesn't separate.

There are two types of emulsion:

OIL-IN-WATER EMULSION

In this emulsion the water is the main phase, with tiny droplets of oil being surrounded by water. This process creates creams and lotions which feel moist but not greasy when applied to the skin and which are absorbed into the skin without leaving much oily residue. A 'vanishing cream' is an example of this type of emulsion.

To make creams and lotions of this type it's necessary to use an emulsifying wax. Many emulsifying waxes come from natural sources such as animal or vegetable fats; others are synthesised in laboratories. If you don't feel comfortable using any synthetics at all then you will have to settle for water-in-oil emulsions.

Oil-in-water Emulsion

PHASE A

Heat the water-phase ingredients to 60°C (140°F), add preservative (if using), stir thoroughly, and continue heating to 70°C (158°F).

PHASE B

Heat the oil-phase ingredients to 70°C (158°F).

Pour the phase A mixture (water phase) in a slow stream onto the phase B mixture (oil phase), stirring constantly. The resulting emulsion should be stirred slowly and continuously until it drops to 45°C (113°F).

PHASE C

Add the other ingredients and mix thoroughly. Pour into sterilised jars and cap immediately.

STEP BY STEP OIL-IN-WATER EMULSION

Heat the phase A ingredients

Heat the phase B ingredients

Add the phase C ingredients and mix thoroughly

WATER-IN-OIL EMULSION

In this emulsion the oil is the main phase and has water packed into it in microscopically small droplets. This type of emulsion forms a cream or lotion which feels oily when first applied to the skin. Most creams containing beeswax, cocoa butter and coconut oil are water-in-oil emulsions and have a greasy 'feel', which largely disperses as the cream is massaged into the skin.

In the recipes you will find that both types of emulsions are dealt with in separate phases and it's important to deal with the phases in the order specified otherwise your emulsion might 'break' (separate).

You will notice that for each recipe the oil contents (waxes, oils, lanolin) are heated separately from the water content (water, herb extracts, glycerine, juices, borax, preservative). It's important to use a double boiler to avoid overheating or burning in the wax phase.

In the final phase, essential oils, tincture of benzoin and other ingredients are added when the mixture has cooled to between 40°C and 48°C (104°F and 118°F). (Perfume and other properties are lost if the temperature is any higher.)

Note: If you are using a stearic acid emulsifier it will not be possible to reduce the pH below 6.5 or 7 or the emulsion will break.

Water-in-oil Emulsion

PHASE A

Melt the phase A hard waxes until liquid but not overheated. Add softer phase A ingredients such as lanolin and dissolve. Add phase A oils very slowly, stopping if the wax begins to solidify. Heat only enough to keep the mixture liquid.

PHASE B

Gently heat the phase B ingredients and add slowly in a trickle to the phase A mixture, stirring constantly and stopping if the mixture begins to solidify. Heat slightly until all is once again liquid.

PHASE C

Add the phase C tinctures and essential oils to the emulsion when the emulsion is below 45–48°C (113–118°F). Mix in thoroughly and when all is a homogenous mass, pour into sterilised jars and cap immediately.

STEP BY STEP WATER-IN-OIL EMULSION

Heat the phase A hard waxes until liquid

Add the heated phase B ingredients slowly in a trickle to the phase A mixture

Add the phase C tinctures and essential oils, mixing in thoroughly

MAKING A HERB OIL BASE

A herb oil base is used in ointments, massage oils, bath oils and creams. There are two methods of making herb oils. One involves heating the oil to 45–48°C (113–118°F); the other uses sunlight only. The first method is the most reliable unless you live in a part of the world which has long periods (at least a week) of hot sunlit days.

I use a crock-pot and the hot method as I find it to be very reliable and trouble free.

Herb Oil Base—Cold Method

The hot method tends to lose a lot of the natural perfume of the plant material while the cold method retains more of the scent.

1 Cover flowers or leaves with a slightly warmed, delicate, scentless oil such as grapeseed or almond. Cover closely.

2 Put in a sunny spot for 1 week.

3 Repeat as for stage 6 above until the oil smells as strongly as you desire.

4 Strain well through double cheesecloth and follow stage 7 in Hot Method, opposite.

STEP BY STEP HERB OIL BASE

When making a Herb Oil Base using the cold method, cover flowers or leaves with a slightly warmed, delicate, scentless oil

When making a Herb Oil Base using the hot method, place the flowers or minced herbs in a double boiler or crock-pot and cover with oil

For both methods, strain the finished oil through double cheesecloth into a jar

Herb Oil Base—Hot Method

This method will make a triple strength oil.

1 Place the minced herbs in a crock-pot or double boiler and cover with oil.

2 Add 1 tablespoon cider vinegar to each litre (32fl oz) of oil, and stir well. Cover with a lid and leave for 1–2 hours. The vinegar extracts properties left behind by the oil and also helps to speed up the extraction.

3 Keeping the cover on, heat gently to no more than 45–48°C (113–118°F); if the oil overheats you will lose some of the important volatile properties of the herbs. When the temperature is reached, turn the heat off and allow to cool.

4 Repeat stage 3 several times over a period of 24 hours.

5 Strain the oil through cheesecloth, squeezing the bag to extract as much oil as possible. If you want a single strength oil you can go to stage 7.

6 To make triple strength oil you need to repeat stages 1–5 twice more, using the original oil each time but topping up with fresh oil to keep the quantity the same.

7 Pour the finished oil into a jar. After a few days you will see sediment at the bottom of the jar. Carefully decant the oil into a clean jar, leaving the sediment behind. Refrigerate the oil until needed. I refrigerate the sediment and use it in packs and masks.

MAKING HERB VINEGARS

Herb vinegars may be used as deodorants, hair rinses, skin tonics, wound washes and bath additives. Choose the herbs suitable for the condition. If using dried herbs, reduce the amount to 30g (1oz).

Herb Vinegar

2 cups (500ml/16fl oz) cider vinegar
60g (2oz) fresh herbs
1 tablespoon glycerine

Heat half the vinegar to just below boiling point. Meanwhile, chop or mash the herbs very finely. Add them to the hot vinegar. Pour into a jar and leave for a week. Strain through double cheesecloth into a clean bowl. Add the remaining vinegar and glycerine and mix well. Pour into a sterilised bottle. This keeps well without refrigeration except in very hot weather.

MAKING INFUSIONS

Infusion is another name for a tea and is made in the same way. It is probably the simplest and most widely used herbal preparation. Infusions are made from the parts of the plant which readily release their aromatic and water-soluble principles in boiling water—for instance, ground seeds, roots and bark, and finely chopped leaves and flowers. Infusions will keep in the refrigerator for 1 or 2 days only.

The recipes in this book refer to single, double and triple strengths of infusions. For example, for drinking, one would normally use a single strength infusion; for hair rinses, facial washes, douches and baths a double strength infusion would usually be suitable; and in ointments, creams and compresses, a triple strength infusion would be stronger and have more effect. Solutions above triple strength usually become saturated so there is no benefit to be gained by continuing the process further.

Single Strength Infusion

It is imperative that a cover be placed on the pan or pot as soon as the boiling water has been added or the essential oils will evaporate off immediately. When a lid is placed on the pan, the oils which are carried in the steam will cool on the lid and drop back into the infusion.

Pour 1 cup (250ml/8fl oz) of boiling water over 2 heaped teaspoons finely chopped fresh herbs or 1 heaped teaspoon crumbled dried herb. Cover immediately and stand for 5–10 minutes; strain before using.

DOUBLE AND TRIPLE STRENGTH INFUSIONS

Double or treble the amount of herbs used in the single strength infusion. Make as for the single strength infusion.

MAKING DECOCTIONS

Decoctions are used in the same way as infusions. Some plants or parts of plants need to be simmered to extract their properties. Roots, barks and whole seeds are the parts usually treated in this way. The material should be chopped as finely as possible. If the pieces are too large, they will need to be well bruised (tapped with a pestle or rolling pin) to free and allow the principles to dissolve into the water.

Single Strength Decoctions

To each 1 cup (250ml/8fl oz) of cold water, add 2 teaspoons fresh or 1 teaspoon dried herb. Bring to the boil, cover tightly and simmer gently for 10–30 minutes depending on the fineness of the material.

Strain and make up to the original 1 cup (250ml/8fl oz) with freshly boiled water.

DOUBLE AND TRIPLE STRENGTH DECOCTIONS

Double or treble the amount of herbs used in the single strength decoction. Make as for single strength decoction.

An assortment of equipment needed to make infusions and decoctions

MAKING MUCILAGES OR GELS

Gels will keep for only a few days even if refrigerated. In order to make a longer lasting gel a preservative should be used.

ACACIA OR GUM ARABIC

Acacia used alone forms a viscous but not gelled preparation and so is best used in conjunction with tragacanth. The powder dissolves slowly in water and makes a gentle, emollient gel.

AGAR-AGAR

This setting agent is derived from seaweed and is available as powder, strands or flakes. It has the advantage of not needing refrigeration in order to form a gel, even on very hot days. Only half the amount of agar-agar is needed compared to gelatine but the resulting gel has a different consistency—experiment to find which you prefer.

Agar-agar Gel

As agar-agar sets quickly, it should be boiled in the whole amount of liquid specified in the recipe and the remaining ingredients should be added before the mixture cools to 27°C (80°F).

A stiffish, clear gel is formed by boiling 1 part agar-agar in 5 parts water. Try a small amount as an experiment (don't forget to keep notes!).

IRISH MOSS GEL

An emollient gel which is very easily made.

Quickly wash 15g ($\frac{1}{2}$oz) Irish moss in a little water. Drain. Place in a small saucepan with 1 cup (250ml/8oz) distilled water to cover. Soak for about 12 hours.

Cover the pan and simmer gently for about 5–10 minutes. Strain through double cheesecloth.

ARROWROOT GEL

This gel may be made as thick or as thin as you require. Try the following recipe first and you will be able to gauge future recipes from the results.

Slowly mix 1 teaspoon powdered arrowroot with $\frac{1}{3}$ cup (80ml/$2\frac{2}{3}$fl oz) cold water in a small saucepan. Stir continuously over a very low heat until the mixture becomes transparent and thick. Remove from the heat. If at this time the gel is thicker than you need, cold water may be slowly mixed in while stirring until the desired consistency is reached.

PECTIN GEL

Pectin is an acid made mainly from the skins of apples. It's lovely for the skin as it has almost the same pH. I understand that the following method may be used to make pectin gel. I haven't tried it but I imagine that the apples would need to be very sour and very underripe.

Barely cover the finely chopped peel of tart windfall apples with water in a saucepan. Simmer for about 1 hour. Strain into a bowl, discard the peel. Return the liquid to the saucepan, simmer the liquid until reduced to at least a quarter. Remove from heat. This concentrate should become a gel when cool.

Pectin Powder Gel

Pectin powder is my preferred gelling agent but bought pectin powder is difficult to mix in water without going lumpy. I have found the following method to work perfectly.

Gradually mix 1 teaspoon of pectin powder with 1–2 teaspoons vodka. Slowly add $\frac{1}{3}$ cup (80ml/$2\frac{2}{3}$fl oz) lukewarm water while stirring gently. Leave to thicken. Add more water if a thinner gel is required.

Note: If the pectin is being used with gelatine, the two powders may be mixed together and sprinkled over very hot water, stirring until dissolved.

MALLOW ROOT GEL

This jelly is wonderfully soothing and may be incorporated into creams, lotions, ointments, baths, shampoos, face washes and baths.

Soak finely chopped mallow root in warm water to cover for about 2 hours. (Don't boil the root because the mucilage becomes solid in boiling water.)

STEP BY STEP PECTIN POWDER GEL

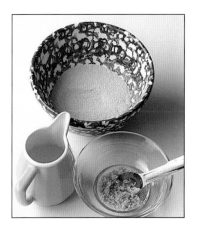

When making pectin powder gel, mix the pectin with vodka first

Slowly add the lukewarm water

Leave to thicken

QUINCE GEL

Simmer 15 fresh quince seeds with $\frac{1}{2}$ cup (125ml/4fl oz) distilled water in a small covered saucepan for 15–20 minutes. Stir often. Strain. Make up to $\frac{1}{2}$ cup (125ml/4fl oz) with more distilled water and allow the mixture to cool and thicken. (Save the seeds as they may be used more than once.)

TAPIOCA GEL

Tapioca is a farinaceous substance extracted from cassava. The gel is soothing, moisturising and demulcent.

Mix $1\frac{1}{2}$ teaspoons tapioca with $\frac{1}{3}$–$\frac{1}{2}$ cup (80–125ml/$2\frac{2}{3}$–4fl oz) boiling water or herbal infusion. Simmer, covered, until the tapioca becomes transparent and soft. Stir often to prevent sticking. Strain through cheesecloth and allow to cool.

TRAGACANTH GEL

Even though tragacanth is expensive it is very useful for making gels. Tragacanth is at its most absorbent when the pH of the mixture is 5.0 (ideal for the skin). Raising or lowering the pH will reduce the viscosity and also the keeping qualities of the product.

METHOD 1
Mix the tragacanth with a little glycerine before adding the water. Add the water very quickly while stirring vigorously.

METHOD 2
Sprinkle the tragacanth powder over the liquid, cover and leave for 24 hours, stirring occasionally.

CAUTION
Inhalation of tragacanth powder can be very dangerous because it swells when mixed with moisture.

MAKING OINTMENTS

Ointments, salves or unguents—as they are sometimes called—are usually a water-in-oil emulsion combined with herbs and used for healing. I'm sure that you, like me, will derive a great deal of pleasure from making ointments. I get a strong feeling of a connection with the herbalists and witches of centuries ago who made these simple preparations in much the same way as I describe.

I make quite a ceremony of the herb collection, choosing a warm and sunny morning and watching for the last drops of dew to dry on the leaves and petals of my chosen plants. I carry a basket and Japanese scissors which I have used for years; secateurs feel too crude for this delicate process! I only collect the amount of herb that I can use immediately.

The tricky part of ointment making is knowing when to pour it into the jar. If you pour too soon the emulsion might break; too late and the mixture won't pour. The following recipe makes 2 x 50g (1²⁄₃oz) jars but it's much easier to make a larger quantity. Jars of ointment are never wasted as they will keep for months in the refrigerator and make excellent gifts.

Basic Method for Ointment Making

½ cube (7g/¼oz) beeswax
30g (1oz) lanolin
¼ cup (60ml/2fl oz) herb oil
2 teaspoons herb tincture
½ teaspoon tincture of benzoin
10 drops essential oil

Melt the beeswax in a small saucepan over a low heat. Add the lanolin and melt. Add the herb oil slowly while stirring.

Take the pan off the heat and cool slightly. Add all the remaining ingredients, stir until the mixture thickens slightly. Pot at once in clean jars.

Ointments are often water-in-oil emulsions with the addition of herbs

MAKING TINCTURES

The undiluted alcoholic tincture made from a single plant is called 'Mother Tincture'—a name coined by Samuel Hahnemann, the founder of homeopathy. In homeopathy the Mother Tincture is diluted by a grinding process (called 'trituration') with either a solid (usually lactose) or a liquid (usually alcohol). A small amount of this mixture is then diluted tenfold, the procedure is repeated and so on. The resulting solutions are referred to as 'potencies'.

If the substance is soluble, a process called 'succussion' is used and this is the process described in Tincture 2: Roots, Bark and Seeds. Tinctures are stronger and more concentrated than infusions or decoctions. They also have the advantage of a long storage life—as much as several years if made with pure alcohol and carefully stored.

To make the tinctures you will need 60–75% proof alcohol, as it is generally a better solvent for plant materials than water and is also a preservative. The keeping quality of the tincture is largely dependent on the strength of the alcohol used. If you are fortunate enough to obtain 95% pure alcohol from a pharmacist you will need to dilute it to 60% using purified water.

Brandy or vodka are excellent substitutes for pure alcohol. Good vodka is about 60% proof, colourless, odourless and tasteless. Obviously, cost is a factor when using vodka or brandy but tinctures may be made in quite small amounts.

Tinctures may also be made from cider vinegar or wine. They won't have the keeping qualities of those made with stronger alcohol, and don't make as powerful a tincture, but are cheap and easy for short-term usage (up to 6 months if stored in the refrigerator).

Tinctures made with vodka and essential oils may be used as colognes or toilet waters. One teaspoon of tincture is equal in strength to 1 cup (250ml/8fl oz) infusion and may be added to poultices, fomentations, compresses, ointments, wound washes or anywhere you want to increase the strength of a remedy. Tinctures such as calendula may be used undiluted where needed to halt infection or to stop bleeding.

Many tincture methods suggest that it's best to determine the amount of herb used by its weight. Over many years I have found that volume is a much more reliable and accurate way. For example, 125g (4oz) of heavy root is a small amount while 125g (4oz) of petals is a large amount and can't be covered by the quantity of alcohol specified.

By following the methods below you will make a very fine tincture.

Tincture 1: Leaves and Flowers

Loosely fill a jar with fresh, finely chopped herb—half fill the jar if using dried herbs. Cover with alcohol and close the jar with a well-fitting lid.

Tincture 2: Roots, Bark and Seeds

Chop finely and bruise 15–30g (½–1oz) herb (amount depends on density). Cover with 1 cup (250ml/8fl oz) alcohol.

Mark the jar (not the lid) with the common name and Latin name of the plant and the date 2 weeks hence when the tincture will be ready.

Keep the tincture where you can see it as it's important to 'succuss' it twice a day. To succuss, put a folded cloth on a workbench and tap the base of the jar gently but firmly on the cloth for about a minute. This releases the properties from the herb into the alcohol.

After two weeks the tincture is ready to strain through a cloth and then through a coffee filter into a dark glass bottle. Label the bottle with the common name, Latin name and the symbol denoting that it is a full strength Mother Tincture.

Store the bottle in a cool dark cupboard (not in the fridge) and it should last for years. If you add 1 teaspoon of glycerine to each 1 cup (250ml/8fl oz) of tincture, the keeping quality is further enhanced.

Fresh or dried herbs and flowers can be used to make tinctures

SKIN AND BODY CARE

I often hear people say 'I don't have time or money to

spend on myself'. We have been conditioned to feel that

time or money spent on nurturing ourselves is 'selfish'. The

end result of this outlook is that one either feels a martyr

(these are revolting people to live with!) or, from expending

too much energy on other people, one becomes so exhausted

that there is no energy left for anyone at all (this is a

dangerous situation which can lead to ill health).

Tablecloth from Linen and Lace of Balmain; flowers by Lisa Milasas

SKIN AND BODY ROUTINE

In a very busy lifestyle, your own 'personal space' time may have to be very carefully rearranged to include some of the following suggestions in your daily routine. (It's said that resistance to change is a sign of aging, so changes in routine could benefit both you and all the people around you!)

A checklist such as the following one helps you to assess your needs, make a plan and determine the amount of time for which you will need to 'budget'. It's useful to keep a note of these needs and plans in a little book.

➤ Are you stressed and have a need to meditate and/or relax? (Time: 15 minutes morning and/or evening.)
➤ Which part of your body is most neglected: feet, hands, face, hair or the whole lot? (Time: 5–10 minutes a day and one morning a month.)
➤ Do you need more exercise? If so, what type? (Time: Daily.)
➤ Do you need to lose weight? (Time: Ongoing but be gentle, realistic and non-judgmental.)
➤ How can you rearrange your life to take the time you need?
➤ What are you going to do for yourself; when and in what order? Time spent meditating, giving yourself a luxurious bath, a hair treatment, a pedicure or a facial is time which will benefit yourself, your family and friends as you will have a more positive outlook and more energy to share. You deserve to give yourself this personal time which is absolutely necessary for your morale and mental, physical and emotional well-being. It helps to make you into a happy person who can cope with the 'ups and downs' of life.

Mothers in particular need this personal cherishing as they spend so much time ensuring that their families are well cared for and happy that they often overlook their own needs.

Try to do something nice for yourself every single day. (See 'Time out'). Money need not be a worrying factor in your body care plans. Most of the ingredients and equipment needed for the simple recipes in this book are already in your refrigerator or kitchen cupboards. If you want to make lots of products to give as gifts or to keep a large family supplied you might have to outlay a little on ingredients or equipment, but the fact remains that you could go to your kitchen now and make something wonderful with ingredients already in the garden, fridge and pantry.

THE NATURE OF SKIN

Skin is a good indicator of the condition of your health. Lack of sleep, inadequate diet, stress and ill health very quickly have an effect and skin becomes a poor colour and texture with lines developing.

I have heard it said that skin is there to 'stop us fraying round the edge', but skin is also the largest organ in the body. Given the right conditions, it is responsible for excreting a third of the waste products from our bodies, so relieving the kidneys of a lot of work.

Our total skin cover measures approximately six metres and weighs between three and five kilograms. It has many layers and is thickest on the back, soles of the feet and palms of the hands. The thinnest skin is found on the eyelids. This wonderful, adaptable, long-suffering covering protects us from the environment, germs and viruses, regulates body temperature and produces hormones and enzymes. Skin is strong and elastic.

Soap dish from Crabtree & Evelyn

A selection of beauty products used in a skin a body routine

It absorbs oxygen, expels carbon dioxide and rejects impurities and toxins.

The skin has three layers: the epidermis, dermis and subcutis.

The epidermis is divided into three layers of its own. The top layer is our barrier against the environment. It is impermeable to any but the finest particles and the pH of this layer is slightly acidic (round about 5.0) which acts as a protection against bacteria.

The bottom layer of the epidermis makes the new cells which, over a two-week period, move through the middle layer and become the top layer where they are shed. This top layer is 'dead' skin which needs to be gently but thoroughly and regularly removed.

The bottom layer of the epidermis also contains cells which produce melanin. This is the pigment which gives the colour to your skin, so those with darker skin have more melanin than fair-skinned people. Melanin acts to protect you by absorbing the sun's damaging ultraviolet rays. This protection is only partial, as shown by the high incidence of skin cancer and premature ageing in hot countries such as Australia, where a high proportion of the population is fair-skinned.

The dermis, which lies under the epidermis, is the layer which contains the 'elastic' fibres, collagen and elastin (cosmetic manufacturers spend millions of dollars promoting the fallacy that their 'miracle' products containing collagen and elastin will replace these proteins in the skin). The dermis also houses the nerve endings, hair follicles, ducts of the sweat glands, and oil glands; and carries the blood vessels (which come from inside the body and are responsible for feeding and oxygenating the epidermis).

The subcutaneous layer of skin lies below the dermis and contains the sweat glands and the fat layer which protects our skeleton and internal body organs.

The openings of the sweat glands on the surface of the skin are called pores. The size of the opening or pore is difficult to change but regular use of toners and astringents can help to give the impression of much finer skin.

The oil in the skin is called sebum. Its role is to protect the skin from the drying effects of wind and sun and to also lock in the natural moisture of the skin. The sweat produced by the sweat glands effectively reduces body temperature as it evaporates on the surface of the skin. The sweat also carries waste products from the body—it is important to bathe or shower regularly to help your body get rid of this waste matter and dead skin. The load on our other excretory organs (liver, lungs and kidneys) is lessened when we encourage our skin to work efficiently.

The condition and type of your skin may change from season to season or even from day to day. Women often find that their skin and hair are different before, during and after menstruation, and there are profound changes during puberty and pregnancy. We need to be aware that 'experts' who tell us that we have a particular type of skin can only make a judgment based on what they are seeing at that moment. We will always be the best judges of our own skin, hair and bodies but sometimes need some encouragement and guidelines to give us confidence.

The very discouraging and demoralising pressure on women to strive for a youthful appearance has resulted in many women going to extreme lengths to try to achieve this.

Plastic surgery is painful and expensive and the results are often disastrous or at best very short lived. Cosmetic manufacturers are amongst the most guilty perpetrators of this 'young is the most beautiful' myth as they stand to make millions of dollars each year from people who are looking for the 'magic potion' which will get rid of wrinkles and keep the taut, smooth skin of an eighteen-year-old. There is, however, a difference between a face which is etched gently and beautifully with the lines of wisdom and laughter and the lined, dried-up, prematurely aged skin of the 'sun-worshipper'.

In the past, fair-skinned women went to great lengths to prevent the sun colouring their skins and destroying their 'peaches and cream' complexions. Sadly, at some stage, suntans became fashionable and, despite well-publicised warnings, many people still cling to the idea that a tan is beautiful.

We all need a certain amount of sunlight each day for stimulating the production of vitamin D and for the metabolism of calcium. This can be safely achieved by taking a ten-minute walk or watering the gardens in early morning or evening sunlight. The ageing process caused by overexposure to sunlight is irreversible and I have seen girls of nineteen and younger with more lines, broken veins and 'liver spots' than a fifty-year-old who has protected her skin and avoided excessive sunlight.

SKIN TYPES

All skins are not the same. As babies we usually have perfect skin: smooth, close-textured, moist, plump and with enough oil to protect but not cause a problem. As we get older the conditions under which we live and our age begin to change the texture of our skin; we need to know how to care for our very individual type in order to keep it as close to baby skin as possible.

The following is a list of the four main skin types and how to recognise and treat them.

NORMAL SKIN

Fairly rare. Normal skin is fine-textured, smooth and soft with no large pores, blackheads, spots, flakes or broken veins apparent. If a tissue is pressed to this skin first thing in the morning there will be only a trace of oil showing. If you are blessed with this type of skin you are among the fortunate few and should take great care of it. Protect it from wind, sun and dry air by using light moisturisers, cleansers and toners.

OILY SKIN

If a tissue is pressed to the face first thing in the morning it will show quite a lot of oil. The texture of the skin is coarse with large pores and a tendency to blackheads and spots due to excessive sebum blocking the pores. The bonus of having oily skin is that it has less tendency to wrinkle than any other type and will get less oily as you get older. It's a mistake to use harsh soaps and strong astringents containing lots of alcohol in an attempt to control excessive oiliness, as these tend to stimulate the skin to produce more sebum and in the long run make the situation worse. Oily skin needs an oil-free moisturiser except on the areas around the eyes, throat and lips where a richer moisturiser is needed. This type of skin benefits from regular use of masks and steams to help unblock pores and prevent blackheads from forming.

COMBINATION SKIN

This type is a combination of normal/dry and oily skin. Press a tissue on your face first thing in the morning—if there is a greasy 'T' shape on the tissue this will indicate combination skin. There may be a tendency to blackheads around the nose and pimples on the forehead or chin. There are often small greasy areas on the jawline.

The programme for this skin has to be oily/normal or oily/dry.

DRY SKIN

Dry skin is fine-textured, delicate and thin with a tendency to line easily. I have skin of this type and rarely use soap and water on my face as it makes my skin feel tight enough to 'crack'—very uncomfortable!

Masks and steams need to be used with great care as they could encourage 'broken' veins to which this type of skin is prone. Night creams, cleansers, toners and moisturisers should be emollient and gentle.

HERBS AND TREATMENTS
FOR SKIN AND BODY

DRY SKIN HERBS

Acacia flower
Aloe vera leaf
Burdock root
Calendula flower
Chamomile flower
Clover flower
Comfrey leaf, root
Elderflower flower
Fennel seeds
Heartsease flower
Irish moss
Lemon grass leaf
Liquorice root
Mallow root, leaf
Nettle leaf
Orange blossom
Orange peel
Orris root
Parsley leaf
Rose petals
Rosemary leaf
Violet leaf, flower
Yarrow leaf, flower

DRY SKIN OILS

Almond
Apricot
Castor
Cocoa butter
Olive
Palm
Peanut

DRY SKIN (MISC.)

Almond meal
Arrowroot
Buttermilk
Cider vinegar
Cream
Dried milk
Egg yolk
Glycerine
Honey
Irish moss
Lanolin
Milk
Oatmeal
Rose-water

NORMAL SKIN

Those of you with normal skin
may use most of the herbs, oils
and other ingredients suitable
for dry skin. Avoid overuse of
the richer ingredients such as
olive oil, beeswax and lanolin.

OILY SKIN HERBS

Aniseed
Calendula flower
Chamomile flower
Clary sage leaf
Comfrey leaf, root
Fennel seed
Heartsease flower
Horsetail stem
Kelp
Lavender flower
Lemon grass leaf
Liquorice root
Lovage leaf
Mallow root
Mandarin peel
Marjoram leaf

OILY SKIN
HERBS (CONTD.)

Mint leaf
Nettle leaf
Orange flower
Parsley leaf
Rose petal
Sage leaf
Southernwood leaf
Thyme leaf
Willow bark
Witch hazel bark, leaf, tincture
Yarrow leaf

OILY
SKIN OILS

Almond
Linseed
Soya bean
Walnut
Wheat germ (10% only)

OILY SKIN
(MISC.)

Almond meal
Almond milk
Arrowroot
Bran
Brewer's yeast
Buttermilk
Cider vinegar
Dried skimmed milk powder
Egg white
Fullers earth
Glycerine
Honey
Kaolin
Oatmeal
Yoghurt

ASTRINGENTS

Agrimony
Alum root
Bay
Benzoin gum
Clary sage
Comfrey leaf, root
Cornflour
Lemon, fruit
Lemon verbena
Lemon grass
Myrrh
Persimmon
Rosemary
Rose, red
St John's wort
Strawberry
Tea leaf
Tomato
White oak bark
Witch hazel
Yarrow

DEODORANTS

Alum powder (see Glossary)
Cider vinegar
Lavender oil
Lemon juice
Lovage leaf
Orange peel
Orris root
Patchouli leaf, oil
Rosemary leaf, twig
Sage leaf
Thyme leaf, oil
Vinegars (herbal)
White willow bark
Witch hazel tincture

ESSENTIAL OILS FOR SKIN

FOR DRY SKIN

Benzoin

Chamomile

Carrot

Evening primrose

Geranium

Hyssop

Jasmine

Lavender

Neroli

Patchouli

Rosemary

Rose

Sandalwood

FOR NORMAL SKIN

Benzoin

Chamomile

Carrot

Evening primrose

Geranium

Lavender

Lemon

Jasmine

Neroli

Patchouli

Petitgrain

Rose

Rosemary

Sandalwood

Ylang-ylang

FOR OILY SKIN

Benzoin

Carrot

Chamomile

Evening primrose

Geranium

Lavender

Lemon

Jasmine

Marjoram

Neroli

Petitgrain

Rose

Sandalwood

Ylang-ylang

FOR ACNE

Carrot

Eucalyptus

Evening primrose

Tea tree

Thyme

White willow bark

FOR ECZEMA

Bergamot

Carrot

Chamomile

Eucalyptus

Evening primrose

Hyssop

Lavender

Patchouli

FOR PIMPLES

Carrot

Chamomile

Clary sage

Eucalyptus

Evening primrose

Geranium

Juniper

Lavender

Lemon

Patchouli

Sandalwood

FOR DEHYDRATED SKIN

Carrot

Evening primrose

Geranium

Jojoba

Lavender

Patchouli

Peppermint

Sandalwood

CLEANSERS

Skin needs gentle treatment. The products you use and the way you apply them have a long-term effect. I have seen some people treat their skin as though they are cleaning the top of a grease-baked barbecue. All your movements should be light and gentle—we only have one face and we need to be kind to it!

In an attempt to defy gravity we should use upward movements when applying cleansers (or anything else) to the throat and face.

If you use cosmetics, then you will need a cleanser which will dissolve the mascara, lipstick or heavy foundation. Very hot water and soap will get rid of the make-up but will also get rid of the skin's natural oils, and the heat could cause broken capillary veins. Most soaps are alkaline and can irritate and dry sensitive skin.

Many skins have very little natural lubrication and feel tight and stretched if soap is used as a cleanser. Other skins have quite a lot of oil and don't feel clean or fresh unless soap and water is used, so choose the cleanser which makes you feel the most comfortable.

In the following pages you will find many different types of cleansers. Based on your knowledge of your own skin you will be able to choose the ones most suitable for you.

JELLY CLEANSERS

Jelly cleansers give us the best of both worlds. They use water and a face-wash action but aren't as drying as soaps; they feel gentle and moisturising but aren't as greasy as creams. Jelly cleansers have the added advantage of not needing to be followed by a toner.

The liquid soap mentioned in the recipes is castile and is often scented with peppermint, almond or other herb fragrances. Castile is among the gentlest of soaps. The setting agents are gelatine and pectin powder or tragacanth.

The amount of setting agent used will vary. If the jelly is to be stored in the refrigerator, you will need less. If you live in a hot climate, you need more. Make a small batch initially, using the amounts in the recipe; keep a note of changes (if any) to make to the next batch. You will probably need to use less pectin than tragacanth.

Please consult the note in Making Mucilages or Gels regarding the mixing of pectin and tragacanth before beginning these recipes.

Honey and Peppermint Cleansing Jelly

1 cup (250ml/8fl oz) hot water
2 teaspoons gelatine
1½ teaspoons powdered pectin or tragacanth
1 tablespoon runny honey
½ cup (125ml/4fl oz) glycerine
½ cup (125ml/4fl oz) liquid soap
1 teaspoon tincture of benzoin
1 dropper peppermint oil

Mix the gelatine and pectin or tragacanth together well. Sprinkle over the hot water. Stir until dissolved. Mix all the remaining ingredients together with the gelatine mixture. Stir really well.

Bottle while still warm. Shake occasionally until cold. Massage gently into wet skin, then rinse off thoroughly. Pat dry.

Medicated Jelly Cleanser

1 cup (250ml/8fl oz) hot water
2 teaspoons tragacanth
2 teaspoons gelatine
½ cup (125ml/4fl oz) glycerine
¼ cup (60ml/2fl oz) runny honey
½ cup (125ml/4fl oz) liquid soap
½ dropper clove oil
1 dropper tea tree oil
½ dropper cajuput oil

Mix tragacanth and gelatine together, sprinkle over the water, stirring until dissolved and no lumps remain. Mix remaining ingredients and add to tragacanth mixture. Stir well to mix. Bottle while still warm. Shake occasionally until cool.

Shake gently before use. Massage gently into wet skin. Leave for 2 minutes. Rinse and pat dry.

Home-made cleansers

MILK CLEANSERS

Quickie Milk Cleanser

A good 'quickie' cleanser is milk (full cream for dry skin; skimmed milk for oily skin) wiped on with a cotton wool ball. There is no need to wash the milk off—it won't smell and will leave a natural sheen on your skin.

If you would like to add a little refinement to this recipe you can put a handful of elderflower blossoms and a spoonful of yoghurt into the milk, heat to just below boiling and leave covered for half an hour. Strain and use.

Milk and Honey Cleanser
ALL SKIN TYPES

A quickly stimulating cleanser for all skins. Removes dead skin, oil and grime.

1 teaspoon dried milk
1 teaspoon almond meal
2 teaspoons honey
½ teaspoon rose-water (optional)
3 drops almond oil

Mix all together well. Pat on from the base of the neck up to the hairline (not around the eyes). Massage gently into the skin. Leave 10 minutes. Wash off with warm water.

Almond Milk
ALL SKIN TYPES

This milk is suitable as both a cleanser and a moisturiser. It will keep for only a few days but may be frozen in ice cube trays and defrosted when needed.

1–1½ cups (250–375ml/8–12fl oz) boiling water
60g (2oz) ground almonds

Mix together the water and almonds, cover and leave overnight in the refrigerator. Strain through double cheesecloth. Keep refrigerated.

CLEANSING CREAMS

Olive Cleanser
DRY/COMBINATION/NORMAL SKIN

If you want a white cleansing cream you will need to buy bleached beeswax from the pharmacy. I like the colour obtained from using raw beeswax.

100ml (3⅓fl oz) olive oil
2 cubes (30g/1oz) beeswax
2 tablespoons rose-water
1 teaspoon borax

Melt the oil and beeswax together in a double boiler. Dissolve the rose-water and borax together in a small saucepan. Don't overheat. Add slowly to the wax mixture while stirring. Remove from the heat. Stir until cool or pour into a jar and shake until cold. If a softer cream is preferred, the amount of oil and rose-water may be increased.

Rose Cleansing Cream
DRY/COMBINATION/NORMAL SKIN

This is one of my preferred cleansers which I use in conjunction with Rose Petal Tonic. This cream is an excellent eye make-up remover.

35g (about 1oz) cetomacrogol emulsifying wax
25g Copha (hydrogenated coconut oil)
½ cup (125ml/4fl oz) grapeseed oil
185ml (6fl oz) purified water
5 teaspoons rose-water
10 drops rose geranium oil
10 drops palmarosa oil

Melt the wax, Copha and grapeseed oil together in a double boiler, don't overheat. Remove from the heat. Heat the water and rose-water in a saucepan to the same temperature as the wax mixture. Add the water mixture to the wax mixture slowly, stirring constantly until lukewarm. Add the essential oils and mix in well. Pour into jars and shake until cool.

Cucumber Cleansing Cream

ALL SKIN TYPES

Blend a chopped small cucumber until liquidised, strain and use the resulting liquid. See the Glossary for more about cucumber. To preserve this cream look at preservatives in the Glossary.

1 cube (15g/½oz) beeswax
1 cube(15g/½oz) cocoa butter
¼ cup (60ml/2fl oz) coconut oil
⅓ cup (80ml/2⅔fl oz) sweet almond oil
100ml (3⅓fl oz) cucumber juice
2 teaspoons glycerine
½ teaspoon borax
½ teaspoon tincture of benzoin (optional)
5 drops essential oil of choice

Melt the wax, cocoa butter and oils in a double boiler. Cool to just above lukewarm.

Dissolve the cucumber juice, glycerine, borax and tincture of benzoin (if used) together in a small saucepan. Don't overheat. Cool to the same temperature as the wax mixture. Add the juice mixture very slowly to the wax mixture, stirring until lukewarm. Add the essential oil and mix in thoroughly. Pour into a jar.

OIL CLEANSERS

Quickie Oil Cleanser

Another quick and inexpensive cleanser is hardened vegetable fat such as 'Copha' (hydrogenated, solid coconut oil). This fat dissolves very easily on the skin, is easily wiped off with a tissue and leaves the skin very smooth. A tonic is needed to remove the last traces of grease.

Simple Cleanser

DRY/COMBINATION/NORMAL SKIN

This cleanser uses ingredients you may already have in your refrigerator. It's inexpensive, cleans gently and well and keeps for a long time without preservative if stored in the refrigerator.

40g (1⅓oz) solid vegetable fat (see Glossary)
100ml (3⅓fl oz) coconut oil
100ml (3⅓fl oz) olive oil
10 drops essential oil of choice

Melt the vegetable fat, coconut oil and olive oil together in a saucepan over a low heat. Stir to mix. Allow to cool a little.

Add the essential oil and mix well until beginning to thicken. Spoon into a jar. Store in the refrigerator.

Making the olive cleanser, a simple recipe

Flowers by Lisa Milasas

FACIAL STEAMING

Facial steaming causes the skin to perspire which helps to deep-cleanse every pore; it also loosens dead skin scales and grime on the skin. The heat from the steam increases the blood supply and also hydrates the skin, leaving it looking and feeling softer and more youthful.

Those of you with 'thread veins' on the cheeks need to be careful when steaming. Apply a thick layer of moisture/night cream over the veins and hold the face about 40cm (16in) away from the steam—no closer. Don't steam more than once a fortnight. If your skin is very dry and sensitive, apply a thin layer of honey over the face and throat before beginning; keep about 40cm (16in) between your face and the steam. Don't steam more than once a fortnight.

Normal, combination and oily skins may be steamed as often as twice a week if liked. If your tap water is treated with chlorine it's wise to use purified water or rain water for steaming, or failing this, expose a bowl of water to the air for 24 hours to get rid of the chlorine. The steam from chlorinated water carries chlorine gas—this can be lethal, or at best, very harmful.

In areas where the water is chlorinated it's wise to keep the bathroom door and window open when bathing or showering as the effects of the gas are cumulative and inhalation over a period of time may explain a general malaise from which you may be suffering.

STEAMING INSTRUCTIONS

Have ready a shower cap, a large towel and a heatproof pad for the table:

1 Wash or otherwise cleanse the face. Put the shower cap on.
2 Put ⅓ teacup finely chopped herbs in a saucepan. Cover with 2 litres (3½ pints) cold water and a lid.
3 Bring to the boil and simmer gently for 5 minutes.
4 Put the saucepan on the heatproof mat and remove the lid.
5 Form a tent with the towel over the saucepan and your head.
6 Keep the face about 20cm (8in) away from the steam and bliss out for about 5–10 minutes. By this time all the deep grime will have floated to the surface.
7 Splash the face with cool (not cold) water and finish with a tonic or astringent and some moisture cream.

The following recipes are for 'standard' steams but you can choose your own blends from the chart of Herbs and Treatments for Skin and Body. I like to make a big batch of my favourite blend to have on hand when the urge to steam comes over me or when my face demands it! Use ⅓ teacup of the blend for each steam.

The herbs and citrus peel should be dried and finely chopped or rubbed. Seeds should be dried and crushed and roots dried and either ground or finely chopped. Essential oils may be used either alone or in combination with dried or fresh herbs.

Note: No more than 8 drops of essential oils may be used in 2 litres (3½ pints) boiling water.

Tin basin, jug and timber bath mat from Linen and Lace of Balmain; jar from The Bay Tree; flowers by Lisa Milasas

Preparing for a facial steam

Steaming Blend for Normal and Combination Skins

See Facial Steaming for instructions.

1 teacup fennel leaves and seeds
1 teacup dried lemon peel and leaves
1 teacup dried orange peel and leaves
1 teacup lavender flowers and leaves

Steaming Blend for Dry Skin

See Facial Steaming for instructions.

¼ teacup chamomile flowers and leaves
1 teacup clover
¼ teacup comfrey root (ground)
1 teacup comfrey leaves
1 teacup fennel seeds and leaves
1 teacup violet leaves and flowers

Steaming Blend for Oily Skin

See Facial Steaming for instructions.

1 teacup chopped lemon grass
1 teacup lemon peel and leaves
¼ teacup liquorice root
1 teacup comfrey root and leaves
¼ teacup peppermint leaves

Steaming Blend for Acne, Eczema and Similar Problems

See Facial Steaming for instructions.

1 teacup lavender leaves and flowers
1 teacup fennel seeds and leaves
1 teacup eucalyptus leaves
1 teacup comfrey root and leaves
1 teacup sage
⅛ teacup thyme

SCRUBS

Scrubs and masks may be used by people of any sex and all ages. They may be used for exfoliating, clearing excessive oiliness, refining pores, increasing circulation, nourishing dry skin and improving circulation.

The frequency with which you use scrubs and masks depends entirely on your skin type. If you have oily blemished skin you will be able to use these preparations several times a week, but if your skin is fine and dry it would be wisest to choose only the most gentle treatment and use it maybe once a fortnight. Areas with obvious thread veins should never be treated with masks or scrubs as the additional stimulation could cause a worsening of the condition.

Scrubs may usually be made in bulk, stored in a glass jar in the bathroom and mixed as needed.

FRUIT AND VEGETABLES FOR SCRUBS AND PACKS

APPLE PULP: Slightly acidic; good for delicate skin
APRICOTS, MASHED: Moisturising, soothing, cleansing
ASPARAGUS: Stimulating; dries up pimples
AVOCADO: Deeply penetrating and full of vitamins
BANANA, MASHED: Nourishing
CARROT PULP: Antiseptic; heals pimples and sores
CELERY JUICE: Acts as a toner for tired or aged skin
CUCUMBER: Cooling, soothing, bleaching, healing
FIG PULP: Emollient and cleansing
LEMON JUICE: Diluted for oily skin and freckles
LETTUCE JUICE: Soothes sore, rough skin; helps to clear pimples
ORANGE JUICE: Hydrating for older skins
PEAR PULP: Soothing and cooling on sunburnt skin
PINEAPPLE PULP: An astringent wash for oily skin
POTATO, RAW: Helps clear blemishes and eczema
STRAWBERRIES, MASHED: Slightly acidic, cleansing and luxurious
TOMATOES, MASHED: Good for oily skins
TURNIP, MASHED: Deep cleansing
WATERMELON JUICE: Good for rough skin and deep cleansing

Avocado Scrub

ALL SKIN TYPES

Avocado oil is very nourishing and penetrates the skin very readily; almonds and cornmeal exfoliate and soften the skin and this recipe is gentle enough to use on a daily basis if the almonds and cornmeal are very finely ground.

This scrub needs to be refrigerated and will only last for a few days but it is very quick and easy to assemble a fresh batch if the ingredients such as the almonds are ground in larger quantities, mixed with the cornmeal and stored in a jar in a cool place.

1 teaspoon avocado oil
1 teaspoon finely ground almonds
1 teaspoon fine cornmeal
½ teaspoon cider vinegar
1 drop ylang-ylang oil
purified water

Combine the avocado oil, almonds, cornmeal, vinegar and ylang-ylang oil in a bowl. Mix to a smooth paste with the water as needed.

Massage the scrub gently into the skin, rinse off with lukewarm water and pat dry.

Parsley and Lettuce Scrub

ALL SKIN TYPES

Lettuce and parsley are both excellent for the skin. The following mixture makes enough for 8–10 treatments.

2 tablespoons finely ground bran
3 tablespoons finely ground oatmeal
1 tablespoon powdered soap
1 tablespoon dried parsley, powdered
2 tablespoons dried lettuce, powdered
1 tablespoon dried comfrey leaf, powdered

Mix all the ingredients together. Store in an airtight jar.

Place 1 tablespoon of the scrub mix in a small bowl. Add enough water, milk or yoghurt to form a soft paste and massage gently into the skin using small circular movements. Rinse off with cool water, then pat dry with a soft towel.

Cinnamon and Herb Scrub

OILY/COMBINATION SKIN

Lemon grass or peppermint infusion would be a good choice for these skin types.

The recipe makes enough mixture for about eight treatments. Store the mixed dry ingredients in a jar and mix 1 tablespoon as needed with a herbal infusion.

⅓ teacup fuller's earth or kaolin
⅓ teacup ground rolled oats
1 teaspoon ground cinnamon
herbal infusion (see Chapter One)

To each tablespoon of the scrub mixture, add enough herb infusion to make a soft paste. Massage gently onto the skin for a few minutes, then wash off with warm water.

Yoghurt, Yeast and Sugar Scrub

The yoghurt cleanses and balances skin pH, the yeast stimulates blood supply, and the sugar smooths and exfoliates. This almost 'instant' recipe is sufficient for one treatment. It does not keep.

2 teaspoons yoghurt
1 teaspoon brewer's yeast
1 teaspoon sugar

Mix all the ingredients together in a small bowl and use immediately before the sugar dissolves.

Gently massage onto the skin. Rinse off with lukewarm water. Pat dry.

MASKS

As most of the following masks are made with fresh fruit, vegetables and milk or yoghurt, they should be prepared as needed or kept for no longer than 24 hours in the refrigerator. Many fruits and vegetables make good masks by themselves. You may like to use a thickener to help stop the mashed pulp from sliding off your face.

HOW TO APPLY

Spread the mask over your face and neck (avoid the eye area and be very careful if you have dry skin or 'broken' veins, as the masks may be over-stimulating). Lie down on your bed or in the bath and put cucumber slices or cotton wool soaked in distilled witch hazel on your eyes. Now... relax... let your mind d...r...i...f...t for 15–20 minutes. Wash the mask off in lukewarm water followed by a cool splash. Pat dry and feel the difference.

Basic Mask

A basic mask may be made in advance and stored in an airtight jar ready for mixing.

100g (3⅓oz) fuller's earth or kaolin
2 tablespoons arrowroot or cornflour
1 tablespoon finely ground rolled oats or fine cornmeal
1 tablespoon finely ground almond meal or wholemeal flour

Mix all together and store in a tightly covered jar.

Mix 1 tablespoon of the mixture to a soft paste with honey, fruit juice or pulp; vinegar; yoghurt; egg; oil; a herbal infusion or a decoction.

Spread the mixture over your face and leave it on for 10–15 minutes. Rinse off with lukewarm water and pat dry.

Quickie Honey Mask
ALL SKIN TYPES

A simple honey mask is a stimulating cleanser for all skin types. It can be done very quickly, easily and cheaply. Spread some warm runny honey over your face and very gently begin to tap your skin with your fingertips (as if your are typing) until there is a feeling of 'pulling' (about 2 minutes). STOP tapping and rinse well with coolish water. Pat dry. If you suffer from thread veins avoid this treatment in the affected areas.

Orange and Honey Mask

This is a deep cleanser which leaves the skin feeling soft. If your skin is dry you may apply a thin layer of moisture cream under the mask.

1 egg, beaten
1 teaspoon canola oil
2 teaspoons orange juice
1 drop orange oil
arrowroot to thicken

Mix the ingredients to a paste with the arrowroot. Store in the refrigerator. Use within 3 days.

Spread over the face and leave on for 10–15 minutes. Rinse off with a cool splash and pat dry.

Oat Mask
ALL SKIN TYPES

The following mask may be used every day if you like, as it refines without drying or overstimulating the skin. If you make up a quantity of oats and milk powder and store it in a big jar you will be able to make this mask in double quick time.

1 tablespoon finely ground rolled oats
1 teaspoon dried milk powder
6 drops almond or olive oil
1 drop geranium or lavender oil
warm water to mix

Combine all ingredients together to make a paste.

Spread the mixture over the face, leave for 10 minutes and rinse with lukewarm water. Pat dry.

Relaxing with the Pawpaw (Papaya) Mask

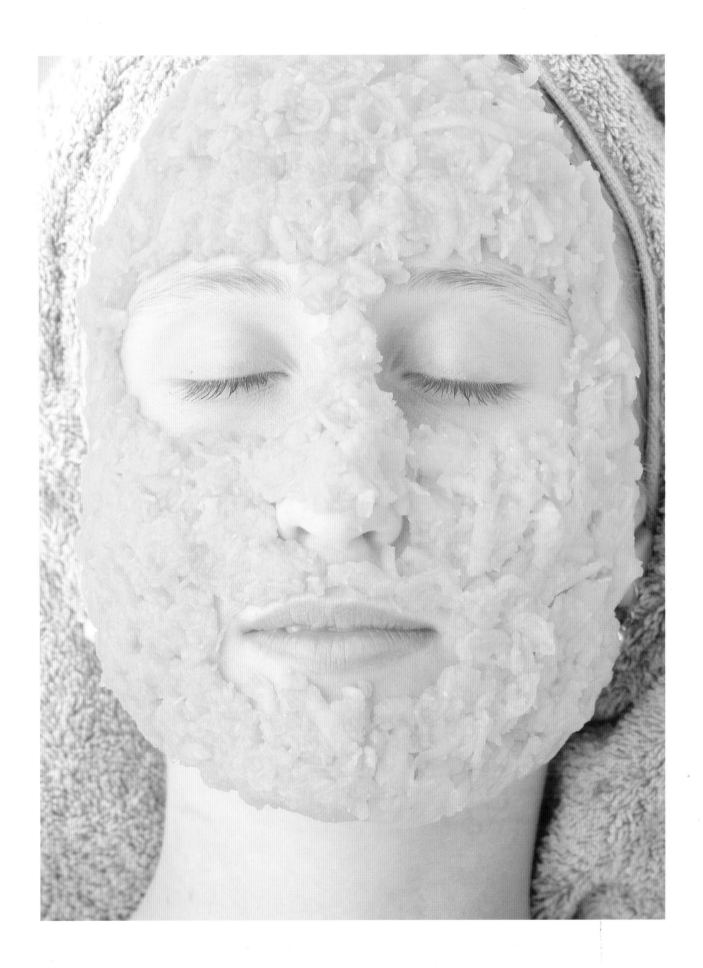

Stimulating Mask

ALL SKIN TYPES

This mask is good for all skin types. If you have thread veins, avoid using the mask on these areas. If your skin is looking sallow and drab you will see a big difference after the ingredients have finished the work of stimulating and cleansing.

1 tablespoon brewer's yeast
2 teaspoons yoghurt
1 teaspoon lemon juice (or orange for dry skin)
1 teaspoon canola or olive oil
1 teaspoon wheat germ oil

Combine all the ingredients together in a bowl.

Spread the mixture over your neck and face and lie on the bed or in a warm bath for 10–15 minutes. Relax. Wash off with lukewarm water and finish with a cool splash. Pat dry.

Quickie Egg Mask

An egg white lightly beaten, smoothed on the skin and rinsed off after 20 minutes will tighten and tone your skin. If your skin is dry you should smear some honey, oil or moisture cream on your skin before spreading the egg white. If you have oily skin, $\frac{1}{4}$ teaspoon lemon juice may be beaten into the egg white.

Pawpaw (Papaya) Mask

OILY SKIN

When you feel that your skin needs a 'spring clean', this is the mask to use. Pawpaw (papaya) contains an enzyme which cleans away the dead cells on the surface of the skin, leaving it soft and fresh. Pineapple contains a similar enzyme and may be substituted.

Mash the pawpaw and spread it over your face, lie down (you won't have any choice as the fruit will run off if you don't get horizontal!), snooze for 10–15 minutes and wash it off with cool water. Pat dry.

Note: Pineapple needs to be blended as it doesn't mash easily.

Oatmeal and Lemon Mask

OILY SKIN

1 tablespoon finely ground rolled oats
2 teaspoons dried skim milk powder
$\frac{1}{2}$ teaspoon lemon juice
warm water to mix

Combine the oats, milk powder and juice in a bowl and stir in enough water to make a paste.

Spread over your face and leave on for 15 minutes. Rinse with lukewarm water and pat dry.

Apricot Mask

NORMAL/DRY SKIN

3 pulped apricots, drained a little
1 tablespoon rose-water
finely ground rolled oats or wholemeal
flour to mix
olive oil

Combine the apricots and rose-water in a small bowl. Add enough oats or flour to make a paste.

Spread a thin film of olive oil on your face then apply the apricot mask. Leave for 10 minutes. Rinse with lukewarm water and pat dry.

Golden Mask

ALL SKIN TYPES

The glow that this golden mask brings to your face is due to the gently stimulating and cleansing action which helps to rid the skin of impurities and to improve sallow complexions.

$\frac{1}{2}$ teaspoon lemon juice
$\frac{1}{2}$ teaspoon orange juice
1 teaspoon carrot juice
1 teaspoon celery juice
1 teaspoon olive oil
1 teaspoon yoghurt
dried milk powder to mix

Mix the juices, oil and yoghurt together in a small bowl. Add enough milk powder to make a paste.

Spread over your face and leave on for up to half an hour for maximum benefit. Rinse off with lukewarm water, then pat dry.

Cucumber Mask

OILY SKIN

1 tablespoon finely grated cucumber flesh
1 tablespoon mashed, cooked carrot
kaolin/fuller's earth or finely ground
rolled oats to mix
1 drop lemon oil

Mix the vegetables together (double the quantities if only using one vegetable). Add enough kaolin or fuller's earth to make a paste which will stay on the face. Add the oil and mix very well. Store in the refrigerator. Use within 24 hours.

Spread over your face and leave on for 15 minutes. Rinse with lukewarm water and pat dry.

'Egg on Your Face' Mask

ALL SKIN TYPES

Egg is a very old, traditional treatment for skin. When combined with milk, yoghurt, oil and honey it becomes a luxury treatment.

1 beaten egg yolk
1 teaspoon honey
1 teaspoon olive oil
½ teaspoon cider vinegar
1 teaspoon yoghurt
dried milk powder to mix

Combine the egg yolk, honey, oil, vinegar and yoghurt in a small bowl. Add enough milk powder to make a paste.

Spread over face and leave on for 15 minutes. Rinse with lukewarm water and pat dry.

Honey, Cream and Almond Mask

ALL SKIN TYPES

Another nourishing and toning mask suitable for everyone. If your skin is very oily you can replace the cream with skim milk. Not only does this mask feel good and make you look good, but it smells good as well.

1 egg yolk
2 teaspoons cream
½ teaspoon runny honey
2 teaspoons fine almond meal
rose-water to mix

Combine all the ingredients together to make a soft paste.

Spread over face and leave on for 15 minutes. Rinse with lukewarm water and pat dry.

STEP BY STEP CUCUMBER MASK

Finely grate the cucumber flesh

Mix the vegetables together

Add enough kaolin or fuller's earth to make a paste, then add the oil

TONICS AND ASTRINGENTS

Skin tonics restore the acid mantle to your skin and leave it feeling fresh and clean. Tonics which contain a large amount of alcohol are called 'astringents'; these can dry the skin as they get rid of all the oil. Even very oily skin can suffer from too frequent applications as the alcohol stimulates the oil glands.

Tonics are made by adding naturally astringent herbs, flowers or citrus peel to vinegar, alcohol, distilled witch hazel or purified water.

Astringents contain the same ingredients but greater quantities of the vinegar, distilled witch hazel or alcohol. A little glycerine may be added to tonics and astringents to counteract any drying effects. These preparations are suitable for pre- and aftershave lotions.

HOW TO APPLY TONICS AND ASTRINGENTS

There are 2 basic methods:

1 Wet some cotton wool with water and squeeze dry (this prevents waste of your precious lotion). Sprinkle with a few drops of the lotion and stroke the cotton wool upwards over your throat and face.

2 Press the damp cotton wool flat and fold in half. Pour on a little toner, hold a corner of the wool and slap your face quite briskly (avoiding the cheeks if there are thread veins). This treatment brings a nourishing, cleansing blood supply flowing to the skin and gets rid of a sluggish, pasty appearance.

SKIN TONICS

Rose-water and Witch Hazel Tonic
ALL SKIN TYPES

Rose-water is one of the gentlest, best known skin tonics. You can buy it from any good pharmacy. Distilled witch hazel is another well known tonic. It is stronger than rose-water and should be tested on a small area before using on dry or sensitive skin. The following is a simple and effective toner for all skins. If your skin is dry you can decrease the witch hazel and increase the rose-water. If you have oily skin you can do the reverse.

100ml (3⅓fl oz) rose-water
¼ cup (60ml/2fl oz) witch hazel
½ teaspoon glycerine

Mix all ingredients together. Pour into a bottle.

Calendula Skin Tonic
ALL SKIN TYPES

A lovely tonic for all skins, particularly those troubled with spots or blemishes. Calendula is among the best known herbs and I use it widely in healing preparations. The benzoin acts as a mild preservative and is also good for skin problems.

1 teacup fresh calendula flowers, chopped
2 cups (500ml/16fl oz) boiling water
¼ teaspoon tincture of benzoin

Mix the flowers and water together in a heatproof bowl. Allow to stand in a warm place for 4 hours. Strain through coffee filter paper.

Bottle and add the tincture. Shake well. Store in the refrigerator.

Calendula Skin Tonic

Elderflower Water

This is a soothing, healing, lotion for the face which has been in the wind and sun and is feeling dry and rough.

1 teacup elderflowers
boiling water to cover
1 teaspoon glycerine
¼ teaspoon tincture of benzoin

Cover the elderflowers with the boiling water in a heatproof bowl. Leave to stand for 6–8 hours. Strain through coffee filter paper.

Add the glycerine and tincture, stir well and bottle. Store in the refrigerator.

Vinegar of the Four Thieves

The archives of the Parliament of Toulouse carry a record concerning the great plague of Toulouse (1628–1631) when a band of four thieves made the most of the opportunity to rob the bodies of the dead and dying. They were reported to be able to avoid infection by washing with herbal vinegar and carrying rags soaked in it. They were finally caught and condemned to be burnt at the stake but this punishment was reduced to one of hanging in return for the disclosure of the secret formula!

Here is what is purported to be the original formula:

3 pints strong white wine vinegar
handful each of wormwood, meadowsweet,
juniper berries, wild marjoram and sage
50 cloves
2oz elecampane root
2oz angelica
2oz rosemary
2oz horehound
pinch camphor

The following recipe is my version of the formula but I have added glycerine for its emollient and preservative properties. One per cent essential oil may be added to the finished vinegar to boost the antiseptic and antibacterial qualities.

This vinegar is useful to help in the prevention of contagious diseases. Rub it on the body, sniff it, spray rooms with it—use it in any way you can when there is a sick person in the house or an epidemic in your neighbourhood.

Vinegar is ideal to use on the skin as it quickly restores the desirable acid mantle. It may be used as follows: aftershave; skin tonic; added to bath water to ease itchy skin; after bath/shower splash; or hair rinse.

2 tablespoons fresh oregano leaves
2 tablespoons lavender flowers
2 tablespoons fresh rosemary leaves
2 tablespoons fresh sage leaves
2 tablespoons fresh mint leaves
1 tablespoon fresh rue leaves
1 tablespoon fresh wormwood leaves
½ teaspoon whole cloves
½ teaspoon ground nutmeg
½ teaspoon ground cinnamon
white wine vinegar to cover
1 cup (250ml/8fl oz) rose-water
2 teaspoons glycerine

Chop all the herbs finely. Put them and the spices in a jar with a tight lid and cover with the vinegar. Cover tightly. Leave in a warm place. Shake often for at least a week. Strain through coffee filter paper. Add the rose-water and glycerine, mix well and bottle.

To make an astringent, dilute a little of the vinegar in the proportions of 1 part vinegar to 8 parts purified water. Keep the remaining vinegar for future use.

Quickie Tonic

A natural mineral water spray (e.g. 'Evian', available from most pharmacies) is a lovely way to cool and moisturise hot, dry skin. I keep a can in the refrigerator so that it's really cold.

When we owned The Prancing Pony restaurant, our skins became very dry while we were working at the stove. The mineral water spray cooled and refreshed us very quickly.

Cucumber Tonic

Cucumbers are cooling and refreshing. The flesh and skin contain different astringencies so use the part most suitable for your skin. The main astringency is in the flesh, so if you have oily skin, peel the cucumber. If your skin is dry or normal, leave the skin on to reduce the astringency.

Cucumber tonic doesn't keep well unless preserved in some manner. If you want to store it for a short time, say 7–21 days, use tincture of benzoin as a mild preservative and keep it refrigerated. If it is for a gift and needs to keep for much longer, you should look at the preservative suggestions in the Glossary.

½ cup (125ml/4fl oz) cucumber juice
½ cup (125ml/4fl oz) distilled witch hazel
1 teaspoon tincture of benzoin

Mix all the ingredients together. Strain through coffee filter paper. Bottle. Store in the refrigerator.

ASTRINGENTS AND AFTERSHAVES

These are much stronger than tonics and are more suited to oily or combination skins. Alcohol is usually included in astringents; if you can't buy pure ethanol you can use vodka, brandy or other high-proof drinking alcohol.

'Spice Islands' Astringent

This delicious astringent smells good enough to drink and is wonderful for oily or combination skins. Men find the spicy perfume pleasing and will use it to freshen the skin after shaving.

1 tablespoon grated orange zest
2 tablespoons chopped fresh peppermint
3 teaspoons mixed spice
1 teaspoon honey
1 tablespoon glycerine
¾ cup (185ml/6fl oz) 70% proof alcohol or vodka
1 cup (250ml/8fl oz) rose water
1 teaspoon tincture of benzoin
4 drops cypress oil
4 drops sandalwood oil

Mix the zest, peppermint, spice, honey, glycerine and alcohol in a jar with a well-fitting lid. Leave in a warm place for a week. Shake often.

Strain through a sieve, then through coffee filter paper.

Add the remaining ingredients, mix well. Pour into a bottle and seal. Leave for 4 days to blend shaking often. Shake before use.

See How to Apply Tonics and Astringents for instructions on use.

Hungary Water

Legend tells that Queen Elizabeth of Hungary was still so beautiful at the age of seventy-two that the King of Poland (don't know how old he was) fell in love with her and proposed marriage. Anyway—here is my version of the astringent she used. I hope it has a similar dramatic result for you!

½ cup (125ml/4fl oz) vodka, brandy or
70% proof alcohol
½ cup (125ml/4fl oz) distilled witch hazel
2 cups (500ml/16fl oz) rose-water
⅓ teacup fresh rosemary leaves
¼ teacup grated orange zest
⅓ teacup grated lemon zest

Place all the ingredients in a jar with a well-fitting lid. Steep for a week, shaking often. Strain well, then filter through coffee filter paper. Bottle.

See How to Apply Tonics and Astringents for instructions on use.

Herbal Aftershave Lotion

This lotion is soothing and healing, it smells good and will give a fresh feeling to your skin.

2 tablespoons finely chopped fresh
calendula flowers
2 tablespoons finely chopped fresh
rosemary leaves
2 cups (500ml/16fl oz) boiling water
50ml (1⅔fl oz) distilled witch hazel
2 teaspoons tincture of benzoin

Mix the herbs and boiling water in a jar and leave for 24 hours in a warm place. Strain through coffee filter paper. Add the witch hazel and benzoin and mix well. Bottle and store in the refrigerator. See How to Apply Tonics and Astringents for instructions on use.

'Pep-up' Astringent

Peppermint leaves skin feeling cool, fresh and clean and the styptic/antiseptic and softening qualities of calendula will take care of any little nicks caused by shaving.

1 teacup fresh peppermint leaves
½ teacup fresh calendula flowers
boiling water to cover
½ cup (125ml/4fl oz) distilled witch hazel
1 teaspoon tincture of benzoin
4 drops peppermint oil

Chop the herbs finely, mix together and cover with boiling water. Leave for 4 hours. Strain through coffee filter paper.

Add the witch hazel and benzoin and mix well. Bottle. Store in the refrigerator.

See How to Apply Tonics and Astringents for instructions on use.

Menthol Aftershave

This leaves the skin feeling cool and clean. It stores well without refrigeration.

¾ teaspoon glycerine
pinch borax
tiny pinch menthol crystals
100ml (3⅓fl oz) distilled witch hazel
5 drops peppermint oil
5 drops sandalwood oil

Put all the ingredients in a 100ml (3⅓fl oz) bottle. Shake several times a day until the borax and menthol are completely dissolved.

See How to Apply Tonics and Astringents for instructions on use.

Shaving mug, brushes, razor and moustache comb from Crabtree & Evelyn

MOISTURISERS

Moisturisers are probably the most advertised skin care products. Manufacturers make extravagant claims which promise that their product will retard or prevent wrinkles and ageing, will 'firm the skin' and even make you look years younger. What a moisturiser will do, if used regularly, is to keep your skin smooth, soft and supple.

The outer layer of your skin is made up of layers of dead scaly cells which need water and oil to keep them moist and supple. Water alone evaporates. Oil alone doesn't soften. Oil and water contained in a moisturiser bind together to hold the water on the skin.

You need a moisturiser if you spend a lot of time out of doors; use air-conditioning; spend time in heated rooms; have normal, dry or irritated skin; are on a drug which is a diuretic; or have eczema or psoriasis.

You will see from this list that almost all people—women, men and children—will benefit from the use of a moisturiser. Dryness accentuates wrinkles; the application of a moisturiser plumps the skin and makes the wrinkles less obvious. Those nasty cracks that can appear on lips, feet and other areas are caused by the severe drying out of the scaly cells which become thick and stiff and then crack. These cracks lead to further drying out from the cells below and eventually an infection could happen.

The main ingredients in a moisturiser are 'occlusive' and 'humectant'. Occlusive ingredients lock in the moisture already present in the skin. Fats and oils are occlusive, with lanolin being one of the most widely used as it closely resembles the sebum in human skin. However, lanolin is an allergen to some people and, if used in too high a concentration, can clog the pores.

Humectants are ingredients which attract water from both the skin and the air. A widely used humectant is glycerine, but if 20% or more glycerine is used it will draw moisture from the skin and into the surrounding air. Humectants loosen dead skin scales and soften hard scales giving the skin a less lined appearance. One may use a single humectant or experiment with a combination of several.

One of the biggest myths promulgated in the advertising of cosmetics is the claim regarding the benefits of collagen and elastin in skin preparations. These two proteins which are manufactured by the body are responsible for keeping your skin elastic and firm. Despite glowing advertisements, these proteins cannot usually penetrate the skin from the outside as the molecules are too large.

The word 'hypoallergenic' doesn't mean that the ingredient or product won't cause allergies. It means that the main allergy-producing ingredients have been replaced or omitted. If you have a super-sensitive skin you would be wise to avoid using the following ingredients in your home-made products:

perfumes (particularly synthetics)
lanolin
vitamin E
paraben preservatives

MOISTURE CREAMS AND LOTIONS

The recipes in this section are mainly emulsions. An emulsion is a mixture of oil and water which, when made, doesn't separate. More care needs to be taken when making this type of preparation as the quantities can be critical.

Very comprehensive instructions for making emulsions, herb oils and infusions will be found in Chapter One.

Always remember that the water phase is added slowly to the oil phase and that essential oils and tinctures aren't added until the mixture is below 45°C (113°F).

If a preservative isn't used, most of the creams must be stored in the refrigerator. For information on preservatives, see the Glossary.

Flowers by Lisa Milasas

Fragrant home-made moisturisers

Elderflower Moisture Cream

DRY/NORMAL/COMBINATION SKIN

This milk-coffee-coloured cream takes quite a time to thicken and always remains fairly soft.

PHASE A

1 cup (250ml/8fl oz) elderflower water

¼ cup (60ml/2fl oz) glycerine

4ml (80 drops) phenoxitol (optional)

PHASE B

25g (⅔oz) cetomacrogol emulsifying wax

5 teaspoons elderflower oil

3 teaspoons castor oil

PHASE C

1 dropper melissa oil

½ dropper clove oil

1 teaspoon tincture of benzoin

Heat the phase A ingredients in a double boiler to 60°C (140°F), add the phenoxitol (if using), stir thoroughly and continue heating to 70°C (158°F).

Mix the phase B ingredients in a separate container and heat to 65°C (149°F).

Pour the phase A mixture onto the phase B mixture in a slow stream stirring gently but thoroughly in a figure of eight motion.

Stir constantly until the temperature is 45°C (113°F). Add the phase C ingredients. Stir for a few minutes to incorporate completely. Pour into sterilised containers and cap immediately.

Extra Rich Cream

DRY AND DELICATE SKIN

This cream is for very dry or mature skin. The smell is redolent of oranges and the colour is orange as well, but don't worry—it won't stain.

PHASE A

150ml (5fl oz) triple strength orange zest infusion

100ml (3⅓fl oz) triple strength mallow decoction

30ml (1fl oz) glycerine

4ml (80 drops) phenoxitol (optional)

PHASE B

20g (⅔oz) cetomacrogol emulsifying wax

2 teaspoons triple strength comfrey/orange herb oil

1 teaspoon sesame oil

1 teaspoon castor oil

1 teaspoon lanolin

½ teaspoon carrot oil (optional)

PHASE C

½ teaspoon orange oil

½ teaspoon clove oil

1 teaspoon tincture of benzoin

Heat the phase A ingredients in a double boiler to 60°C (140°F), add the phenoxitol (if using), stir thoroughly and continue heating to 70°C (158°F).

Mix the phase B ingredients in a separate container and heat to 65°C (149°F).

Pour the phase A mixture onto the phase B mixture in a slow stream stirring gently but thoroughly in a figure of eight motion.

Stir constantly until the temperature is 45°C (113°F). Add the phase C ingredients. Stir for a few minutes to incorporate completely. Pour into sterilised containers and cap immediately.

Cucumber Moisture Lotion

I love this cool, pale green lotion—it can be used on all but the oiliest skins. To prepare the cucumber water, chop unpeeled cucumber, liquidise and strain (through a sieve and then through coffee filter paper).

PHASE A

1 cup (250ml/8fl oz) cucumber water (see above)

3 teaspoons glycerine

4ml (80 drops) phenoxitol (optional)

PHASE B

20g (⅔oz) cetomacrogol emulsifying wax

2 tablespoons almond oil

2 tablespoons avocado oil

1 teaspoon lanolin

PHASE C

2 teaspoons distilled witch hazel

½ dropper lemon oil

½ dropper sandalwood oil

½ dropper tincture of benzoin

Heat the phase A ingredients in a double boiler to 60°C (140°F), add the phenoxitol (if using), stir thoroughly and continue heating to 70°C (158°F).

Mix the phase B ingredients in a separate container and heat to 65°C (149°F).

Pour the phase A mixture onto the phase B mixture in a slow stream stirring gently but thoroughly in a figure of eight motion.

Stir constantly until the temperature is 45°C (113°F). Add the phase C ingredients. Stir for a few minutes to incorporate completely. Pour into sterilised containers and cap immediately.

Calendula Face and Body Lotion

This golden moisture lotion is suitable for the whole family. To make the calendula oil and infusion, see Chapter One.

PHASE A

200ml (7fl oz) triple strength calendula infusion

2 teaspoons glycerine

3ml (60 drops) phenoxitol (optional)

PHASE B

15g (½oz) cetomacrogol emulsifying wax

2 tablespoons calendula oil

PHASE C

20 drops carrot oil

15 drops essential oil

Heat the phase A ingredients in a double boiler to 60°C (140°F), add the phenoxitol (if using), stir thoroughly and continue heating to 70°C (158°F).

Mix the phase B ingredients in a separate container and heat to 65°C (149°F).

Pour the phase A mixture onto the phase B mixture in a slow stream stirring gently but thoroughly in a figure of eight motion.

Stir constantly until the temperature is 45°C (113°F). Add the phase C ingredients. Stir for a few minutes to incorporate completely. Pour into sterilised containers and cap immediately.

Extra-rich Body Lotion

This body lotion is also suitable for face and hands. It's for neglected skin or for sports people or others who spend a lot of time exposed to the elements.

PHASE A

150ml (5fl oz) triple strength herb infusion

100ml (3⅓fl oz) aloe juice

30ml (1fl oz) glycerine

3ml (60 drops) phenoxitol (optional)

PHASE B

15g (½oz) cetomacrogol emulsifying wax

1 teaspoon olive oil

1 teaspoon almond oil

1 teaspoon wheat germ oil

1 teaspoon avocado oil

1 teaspoon lanolin

PHASE C

20 drops evening primrose oil

30 drops lavender oil

20 drops sandalwood oil

1 teaspoon tincture of benzoin

Heat the phase A ingredients in a double boiler to 60°C (140°F), add the phenoxitol (if using), stir thoroughly and continue heating to 70°C (158°F).

Mix the phase B ingredients in a separate container and heat to 65°C (149°F).

Pour the phase A mixture onto the phase B mixture in a slow stream stirring gently but thoroughly in a figure of eight motion.

Stir constantly until the temperature is 45°C (113°F). Add the phase C ingredients. Stir for a few minutes to incorporate completely. Pour into sterilised containers and cap immediately.

Vita-plus Moisture Cream

This is a true 'vanishing' cream which leaves the skin soft but not greasy. It keeps well but in very hot weather the oil content may become rancid if the cream is not refrigerated.

PHASE A

8ml ($\frac{1}{4}$fl oz) glycerine

40 drops triethanolamine

100ml ($3\frac{1}{3}$fl oz) purified water

PHASE B

30g (1oz) stearic acid

1 teaspoon lanolin

1 teaspoon almond oil

1 teaspoon apricot oil

1 teaspoon avocado oil

1 teaspoon wheat germ oil

PHASE C

20 drops essential oil of choice

Heat the phase A ingredients in a double boiler to 60°C (140°F), stir thoroughly and continue heating to 70°C (158°F).

Mix the phase B ingredients in a separate container and heat to 65°C (149°F).

Pour the phase A mixture onto the phase B mixture in a slow stream stirring gently but thoroughly in a figure of eight motion.

Stir constantly until the temperature is 45°C (113°F). Add the phase C ingredient. Stir for a few minutes to incorporate completely. Pour into sterilised containers and cap immediately.

Almond Satin Moisture Lotion

MOST SKIN TYPES

PHASE A

1 teaspoon lanolin

1 cube (15g/$\frac{1}{2}$oz) beeswax

100ml ($3\frac{1}{3}$fl oz) almond oil

$\frac{1}{4}$ cup (60ml/2fl oz) sesame oil

PHASE B

300ml (10fl oz) water

1 teaspoon borax

PHASE C

10 drops essential oil

Melt the phase A ingredients gently in a double boiler, stirring often until the mixture is liquid but not overheated. Mix the phase B ingredients in a separate container and warm to the same temperature as the phase A mixture.

Slowly trickle the phase B mixture into the phase A mixture. Stir constantly and reheat slightly if the mixture begins to solidify.

Add the phase C ingredient when the mixture is 50°C (122°F) or just below. Stir well until no water droplets can be seen. Spoon into sterilised containers and cap immediately.

'Precious Oil' Moisturiser

DRY/NORMAL/DAMAGED SKIN

This is a soft, silky cream which feels luxurious and soothing to the skin.

PHASE A

$\frac{1}{2}$ cube (7g/$\frac{1}{4}$oz) beeswax

$\frac{1}{2}$ cube (7g/$\frac{1}{4}$oz) cocoa butter

$\frac{1}{2}$ teaspoon liquid lecithin

2 teaspoons avocado oil

2 teaspoons olive oil

1 tablespoon almond oil

1 tablespoon apricot oil

PHASE B

1 teaspoon glycerine

2 tablespoons purified water

1 teaspoon borax

PHASE C

20 drops essential oil of choice

10 drops carrot oil

Melt phase the A ingredients gently in a double boiler stirring until the mixture is liquid but not overheated. Mix phase B ingredients in a separate container and warm to the same temperature.

Slowly trickle the phase B mixture into the phase A mixture. Stir constantly and reheat slightly if the mixture begins to solidify.

Add the phase C ingredients when the mixture is 50°C (122°F) or just below. Stir well until no water droplets can be seen. Spoon into sterilised containers and cap immediately.

'Precious Oil Moisturiser'—a soft, silky cream

Flowers by Lisa Milasas

Apricot Rose Cream

DRY/COMBINATION/NORMAL SKIN

A very light cream which glides on easily.

PHASE A

2 tablespoons almond oil

2 tablespoons apricot oil

¼ cube (4g/⅛oz) beeswax

PHASE B

30ml (1fl oz) rose-water

½ teaspoon borax

PHASE C

2 x 250 IU vitamin E capsules

10 drops essential oil of choice

Melt phase the A ingredients gently in a double boiler, stirring often until the mixture is liquid but not overheated. Mix the phase B ingredients in a separate container and warm to the same temperature as the phase A mixture.

Slowly trickle the phase B mixture into the phase A mixture. Stir constantly and reheat slightly if the mixture begins to solidify.

Pierce the vitamin E capsules and add with the essential oil when the mixture is 50°C (122°F) or just below. Stir well until no water or oil droplets can be seen. Spoon into sterilised containers and cap immediately.

NIGHT CREAMS

Night creams are usually much richer and thicker than day creams but it isn't necessary to go to bed with a layer of grease on your face. Skin absorbs as much as it can within 20 minutes of application. Apply night cream while doing the final showering/bathing of the day: the steam will help the cream to penetrate and the surplus may be tissued away before you go to bed.

Don't forget that all skins need extra nourishment and moisture on the throat and round the eyes and the lips.

Honey and Vitamin Emollient Night Cream

DRY SKIN

PHASE A

2 tablespoons lanolin

1 teaspoon honey

2 x 250 IU vitamin E capsules

½ teaspoon almond oil

5 drops carrot oil

½ teaspoon liquid lecithin

PHASE B

⅓ cup (80ml/2⅔fl oz) warm water

PHASE C

6 drops ylang-ylang oil

2 drops sandalwood oil

Pierce the vitamin E capsules and squeeze into the other ingredients in phase A. Melt gently in a double boiler stirring until the mixture is liquid but not overheated. Warm the phase B ingredient in a separate container to the same temperature.

Slowly trickle the phase B ingredient into the phase A mixture. Stir constantly and reheat slightly if the mixture begins to solidify.

Add the phase C ingredients when the mixture is 50°C (122°F) or just below. Stir well until no water droplets can be seen. Spoon into sterilised containers and cap immediately.

'Oranges and Lemons' Night Cream

PHASE A

3 egg yolks

½ teaspoon lemon juice

1 teaspoon orange juice

1 teaspoon glycerine

PHASE B

olive oil to mix

PHASE C

yoghurt to mix

Beat the phase A ingredients in a blender or with a whisk until well mixed. Drizzle the olive oil in very slowly—still beating constantly—until the mixture is very thick. Beat in enough yoghurt to thin to the desired consistency.

Use a night cream to add nourishment and moisture to skin

Timber boxes, photo frames and tablecloth from Linen and Lace of Balmain

EYE CARE

The skin around the eyes is thin, has fewer or no oil glands and is most delicate. Creams must be gentle and soft as must also the feathery touch used to apply them. Use only the best cold-pressed oils and the finest essential oils. The appearance of our eyes suffers from inadequate sleep, poor liver function, lack of exercise, excessive reading or using a visual display unit (VDU) for excessively long periods. If you work at a VDU take your eyes from the display at least every 15 minutes and gaze at the furthest point you can see.

To strengthen and relax the eye muscles, do the following exercise:

Cup the palms over the eyes, excluding all light. Keep the eyes open and look at 'black' for 5–10 minutes. Now press gently, slowly and firmly along the bony edge between the eyes and brows, beginning at the inner edge. Follow the bone around the eyes, under the eyes and at the top of the cheekbone, until you reach the bridge of the nose.

To reduce puffiness: Place cold, used tea bags or chamomile tea over the lids. Or place slices of cucumber or raw potato over the eyes.

Eye Cream

This cream will soften lines around the eyes and help to prevent more from forming. Be persistent—Rome wasn't built in a day!

PHASE A
1 tablespoon lanolin
2 teaspoons almond oil
2 teaspoons wheat germ oil
1 teaspoon apricot oil
PHASE B
2 teaspoons purified water

Melt the phase A ingredients gently in a double boiler, stirring often until the mixture is liquid but not overheated.

Warm the phase B ingredient in a separate container to the same temperature as the phase A mixture. Slowly trickle the phase B ingredient into the phase A mixture. Stir constantly until cool. Spoon into sterilised containers and cap immediately.

Gentle Eye Cream

This is a soft, gentle cream which contains liquid lecithin. It's the best eye cream possible and far superior to any commercial product on the market at the moment. Powdered lecithin isn't suitable. Store in the refrigerator.

PHASE A
1 tablespoon lanolin
1 teaspoon liquid lecithin
2 teaspoons coconut oil
1 tablespoon hazelnut or almond oil
1 teaspoon sesame oil
1 teaspoon avocado oil
PHASE B
2 teaspoons purified water
PHASE C
2 drops lavender oil

Melt the phase A ingredients gently in a double boiler stirring often until the mixture is liquid but not overheated. Warm the phase B ingredient in a separate container to the same temperature as the phase A mixture.

Slowly trickle the phase B ingredient into the phase A mixture. Stir constantly and reheat slightly if the mixture begins to solidify.

Add the phase C ingredient when the mixture is 50°C (122°F) or just below. Stir well until no water droplets can be seen. Spoon into sterilised containers and cap immediately.

*Relaxing with cucumber slices over
the eyes helps to reduce puffiness*

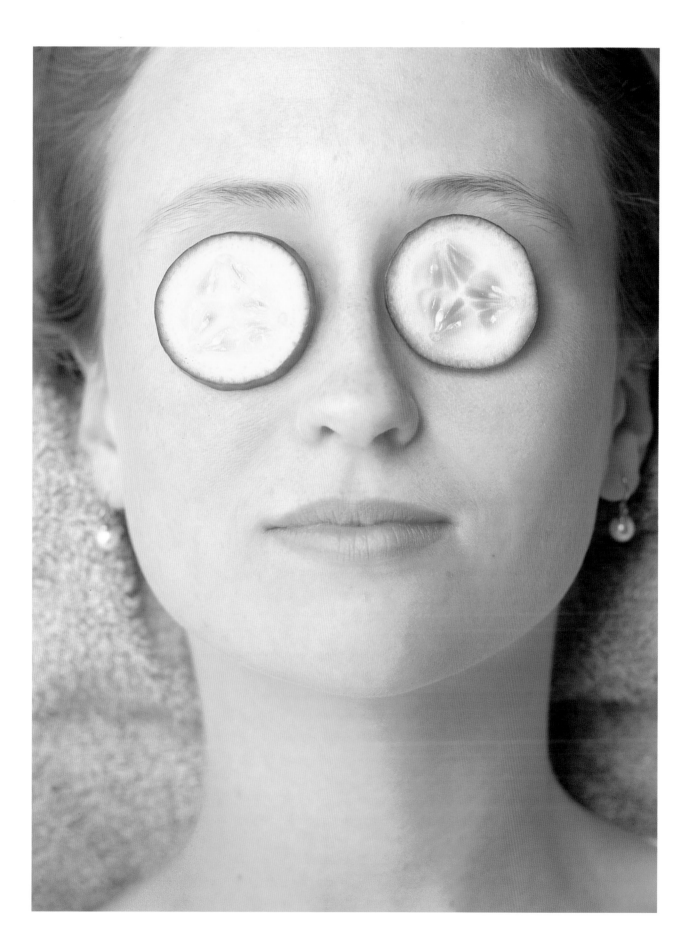

LIP SALVES

Lips should always be kissable but unfortunately are often plagued with cold sores, cracks, lines and dryness. The ingredients in the following lip salve will heal chapped lips and, if used regularly, will prevent further damage.

Soothing Lip Salve

Use this cream at night and during the day if you don't use lipstick. If you don't have cocoa butter, increase the amount of beeswax by half. The amount of oil used will determine the hardness of the finished produce. Glycerine is an important ingredient in this recipe but needs to be very well mixed in or the mixture will separate.

PHASE A
½ cube (7g/¼oz) beeswax
½ cube (7g/¼oz) cocoa butter
PHASE B
¼ cup (60ml/2fl oz) almond oil
5 drops carrot oil
2 x 250 IU vitamin E capsules
PHASE C
½ teaspoon glycerine
4 drops lemon oil

Melt the phase A ingredients gently together in a small saucepan. Add the phase B ingredients and don't overheat. Pierce the vitamin E capsules and squeeze into the mixture.

Beat in the phase C ingredients until completely incorporated. Pot quickly while still soft.

Rosemary Lip Repair

Here is another salve which will both heal and prevent cracks, chapping and dryness of the lips. The sesame oil in this recipe will help to guard against sunburn.

PHASE A
1 cube (15g/½oz) beeswax
PHASE B
2 tablespoons light sesame oil
1 tablespoon wheat germ oil
1 teaspoon almond oil
10 drops rosemary oil
2 x 250 IU vitamin E capsules
PHASE C
½ teaspoon glycerine

Melt the phase A ingredient gently in a small saucepan. Add the phase B oils but don't overheat. Pierce the vitamin E capsules and squeeze into the mixture.

Add the phase C ingredient and beat until no moisture drops are visible. Pot the mixture quickly while still soft.

TOOTH CARE

Regular visits to the dentist, brushing with a medium bristle brush after eating, flossing once a day and eating foods which give both jaws and teeth good exercise, are all sensible precautions to take in order to have strong teeth. If for some reason you aren't able to floss or clean after a meal, eat a piece of cheddar cheese instead—the cheese neutralises mouth acids and is a better choice than a piece of fruit which contains sugar.

There are many alternatives to conventional toothpaste. Most are cheaper and just as effective. Be aware though that harsh abrasives will scratch and damage tooth enamel and, if in doubt, have a word with your dentist before using home-made preparations on a regular basis.

Some of the abrasives which can be used are: heavy magnesium carbonate, calcium carbonate, finely ground cuttlefish bone, finely ground pumice, kaolin powder, bicarbonate of soda and finely ground common salt. The coarsest and harshest abrasives should be very finely ground before use.

Certain dried, powdered herbs, such as sage, act as antibacterial, antiviral/antifungal agents and breath sweeteners when included in toothpowders or toothpastes.

Sage Toothpowder

¼ teacup finely ground sea salt
½ teacup bicarbonate of soda
1 tablespoon dried sage leaves, finely
ground and sieved
1 tablespoon dried peppermint leaves, finely
ground and sieved
10 drops tincture of myrrh

Mix all the dry ingredients. Add one drop of tincture at a time while stirring, to prevent caking. Store in airtight jars. Use a different jar for each member of the family to prevent the spread of any mouth infections.

Cinnamon Toothpowder

1 teacup bicarbonate of soda
2 tablespoons ground sea salt
1 tablespoon dried lemon peel, powdered
1 teaspoon ground cinnamon

Mix all the ingredients together. Store in airtight jars. Use a different jar for each member of the family to prevent the spread of any mouth infections.

Orange Toothpowder

½ teacup calcium carbonate
(precipitated chalk)
½ teacup bicarbonate of soda
10 drops peppermint oil
5 drops cinnamon oil

Mix the dry ingredients in a bowl. Add the oils a drop at a time while stirring, to prevent caking. Store in airtight jars. Use a different jar for each member of the family to prevent the spread of any mouth infections.

Peppermint Toothpowder

This toothpowder does an excellent job. It sweetens and cleans thoroughly, but I think you might need to add some sweetener as the soap makes it rather unpalatable.

1 teacup calcium carbonate
2 tablespoons bicarbonate of soda
1 teaspoon powdered soap
5 drops clove oil
10 drops spearmint oil
5 drops peppermint oil

Mix the dry ingredients together in a bowl. Mix the oils together in a separate bowl and add one drop at a time to the dry ingredients, stirring constantly to prevent caking. Store in airtight jars. Use a different jar for each member of the family to prevent the spread of any mouth infections

MOUTHWASHES

Mouthwashes can be used to freshen the mouth, sweeten the breath, keep bacteria and fungus infections at bay, and ensure the health of gums.

You can also use a plain infusion of herbs for a cleansing mouthwash. Herbs such as the mints, rosemary, lavender, sage, pennyroyal, marjoram and thyme all work very well.

The mouthwashes following have excellent therapeutic qualities.

Quickie Mouthwash 1

A teaspoon of cider vinegar or rose-water in a glass of water will freshen the mouth.

Honey & Mint Mouthwash

Myrrh and honey help to heal mouth ulcers.

½ cup (125ml/4fl oz) brandy/sherry mixed
1 tablespoon cider vinegar
1 teaspoon runny honey
1 tablespoon dried, crushed peppermint leaves
1 tablespoon dried, crushed sage leaves
1 teaspoon ground cloves
10 drops tincture of myrrh

Mix all the ingredients in a jar. Steep for a week, shaking often. Strain well and bottle. Add 1 teaspoon mouthwash mixture to ¼ tumbler water and rinse well.

Sage and Thyme Mouthwash

Thyme is well known for its powerful antiseptic properties. This mouthwash will keep the mouth healthy and sweet-smelling. It will also help to cure sore or ulcerated mouths.

100ml (3⅓fl oz) sherry
100ml (3⅓fl oz) vodka or brandy
1 tablespoon dried crushed thyme leaves
1 tablespoon dried crushed sage leaves
2 teaspoons glycerine
10 drops peppermint oil
10 drops lavender oil
5 drops tea tree oil

Mix all the ingredients in a jar. Steep for a week, shaking often. Strain through coffee filter paper. Bottle. Add 1 teaspoon of mouthwash mixture to ½ tumbler warm water and rinse mouth. Don't swallow the mouthwash.

HAND CARE

We often spend time on our faces but tend to overlook the hands and feet. Wherever there is hair on the body there are sebaceous glands. The hair on the back of the hands and feet is usually sparse, fine and short, and in consequence the glands are also much fewer and the amount of oil produced is insufficient to keep the skin soft and smooth. The combination of this effect and the fact that our hands are subject to more work and physical stress than any other part of our body (and often are given less attention), results, as we age, in loose, wrinkled, blotchy skin. Frequent use of rich cream, the wearing of rubber gloves when washing dishes, gardening and carrying out all the other jobs which stress the skin, will help to keep hands soft and smooth or restore those already work-worn. The benefit of a little attention shows very quickly.

Hand Cleanser

This simple hand cleanser is very thorough but gentle. It will remove soil and grease very efficiently.

60g (2oz) finely powdered soap
60g (2oz) fine sawdust
½ teaspoon borax (optional)

Mix all the ingredients together in a bowl. Keep in an airtight container. Put a teaspoonful of the mixture on the palm of the hand, drizzle on enough water to form a paste and work up to a lather. Rinse off and pat the hands dry.

Quickie Lemon and Sugar Scrub

Massage into the hands 1 tablespoon lemon juice mixed with 1–2 tablespoons sugar. Rinse off, pat dry and apply a little of one of the following hand creams. Your hands will feel like smooth satin.

Lemon Hand Cream

This cream whitens and softens even the most work-worn hands if used regularly. It's an oil-in-water emulsion and so is very easy to massage into the hands without leaving a sticky feeling.

Because of the herbal content this cream needs a preservative, or it will deteriorate quickly.

PHASE A
¼ cup (60ml/2fl oz) aloe juice (see Chapter One)
¼ cup (60ml/2fl oz) triple strength lemon grass infusion
1 teaspoon lemon juice, strained
1 tablespoon glycerine
30 drops phenoxitol (optional)
PHASE B
30g (1oz) cetomacrogol emulsifying wax
1 tablespoon lemon peel oil (see Making Herb Oils in Chapter One)
1 teaspoon lanolin
PHASE C
1 teaspoon tincture of benzoin
1 dropper lemon oil
½ dropper sandalwood oil

Heat the phase A ingredients in a double boiler to 60°C (140°F), add the phenoxitol (if using), stir thoroughly and continue heating to 70°C (158°F).

Mix the phase B ingredients in a separate container and heat to 65°C (149°F). Pour the phase A mixture onto the phase B mixture in a slow stream, stirring gently but thoroughly in a figure of eight motion.

Stir constantly until the temperature is 45°C (113°F). Add the phase C ingredients. Stir for a few minutes to incorporate completely. Pour into sterilised containers and cap immediately.

Hand Softener

If your hands are really rough, use this rich cream during the evening while talking or watching television, or massage a goodly amount on before bedtime and cover the hands with cotton gloves.

Both this recipe and the Lemon and Lavender Hand Softener are water-in-oil emulsions and so have a greasier feel. They are, however, far superior if your hands are really dry and rough.

The following makes a larger quantity than most of the recipes, as gardeners, bricklayers and others who work with their hands will always want plenty of this cream available.

PHASE A

1½ cubes (22g/¾oz) beeswax

¼ cup (60ml/2fl oz) almond oil

1 teaspoon castor oil

¼ cup (60ml/2fl oz) olive oil

PHASE B

2 tablespoons glycerine

2 tablespoons water

PHASE C

1 dropper lemon oil

1 dropper lavender oil

Melt the phase A ingredients gently in a double boiler, stirring often until the mixture is liquid but not overheated. Slowly trickle the phase B ingredients into the phase A mixture. Stir constantly and reheat slightly if it begins to solidify.

Add the phase C ingredients when the mixture is 50°C (122°F) or just below. Stir well until no water or oil droplets can be seen. Pot in sterilised containers and cap immediately.

Rose-water and Glycerine

This is an old favourite in a slightly different guise.

1 tablespoon rose-water

2 teaspoons glycerine

½ teaspoon vinegar

½ teaspoon runny honey

20 drops lemon oil

Mix all ingredients together in a 50ml (1²⁄3fl oz) bottle. Shake well.

Lemon and Lavender Hand Softener

PHASE A

2 cubes (30g/1oz) beeswax

100ml (3⅓fl oz) almond oil

½ cup (125ml/4fl oz) canola oil

PHASE B

2 tablespoons glycerine

PHASE C

2 droppers lemon oil

1 dropper sandalwood oil

1 teaspoon tincture of benzoin

Melt the phase A ingredients gently in a double boiler, stirring often until the mixture is liquid but not overheated. Add the phase B ingredient and stir well to incorporate.

Add the phase C ingredients when the mixture is 50°C (122°F) or just below. Stir well until no water or oil droplets can be seen. Pot in sterilised containers and cap immediately.

Honey Hand Lotion

This simple hand lotion is easy to make and use. It will separate on standing and needs to be shaken before use.

1 teaspoon avocado oil

1 teaspoon almond oil

1 tablespoon runny honey

100ml (3⅓fl oz) rose-water

1 teaspoon glycerine

1 tablespoon white wine vinegar

Warm the oils and honey to lukewarm until the honey is melted. Heat the remaining ingredients separately until roughly the same temperature as the oils and honey. Combine both mixtures and beat together until cool. Bottle and shake well. Shake before using.

Applying the Honey Hand Lotion

Hairbrush and soap dish from Crabtree & Evelyn; flowers by Lisa Milasas

FOOT CARE

Feet are the unsung heroes who carry us, more or less uncomplainingly, on our journey through possibly eighty years. We usually give them attention only if they ache or grow corns. We abuse our feet with ill-fitting shoes, synthetic shoes, stockings or socks; by cutting toe nails incorrectly, weighing too much, standing for too long. Let's give a thought and a cheer to the feet and promise them a bit of loving care.

Most of the recipes used for the hands will be suitable for the feet but here are some additional recipes for special problems.

HERBAL FOOT MASSAGE

This treatment is a very special one for feet aching and swollen from standing too long, arthritic feet or for the swelling and weakness after fractures when the plaster has been removed.

Half fill a foot bath large enough for both feet with warm water and put a few round smooth pebbles in the bottom.

Sprinkle 2 tablespoons herbal vinegar (see Herbal Foot Bath) in the water and 4 drops black pepper oil on the surface. Agitate the water.

Put your feet in the water and roll the soles and under the toes on the pebbles, do this for 5–10 minutes as often as you like.

HERBAL FOOT BATH

If your work involves a lot of standing, your feet are probably aching when you get home. Make the following herbal vinegar and use very cold for the most soothing effect. Make a strong herbal vinegar by placing finely chopped bay leaves, lavender, pennyroyal, sage, thyme and rosemary (it doesn't matter if you don't have all of these herbs) in a heatproof jar and covering with very hot cider vinegar. Cover the jar with a lid and leave for 1 week, shaking daily. Strain through coffee filter paper and store in a clean bottle.

Dab the vinegar on the feet and allow to air-dry.

FOOT BATH

This is another soothing treatment for tired and aching feet.

Make enough triple strength infusion/decoction to half fill a bowl large enough for both feet. Use as many of the following herbs as you can: comfrey root, lavender, pennyroyal, pine needles, rosemary, sage, yarrow.

Have the infusion/decoction as hot as you can bear. Have another bowl containing cold water and alternate the feet between the hot and cold water. Soak the feet for a total of 10–15 minutes spending 2–3 minutes each time in the different temperatures. Finish by massageing the feet with a mixture of half water half witch hazel. Pat dry and massage with Herbal Foot Oil.

Foot Powder

This powder may be sprinkled inside socks and shoes if you suffer from sweaty or smelly feet.

1 teacup kaolin powder
1 teacup unperfumed talcum powder
½ teacup ground arrowroot
2 tablespoons dried powdered sage leaves
2 tablespoons dried powdered rosemary leaves
10 drops lavender oil
10 drops tea tree oil
10 drops tincture of myrrh
10 drops tincture of benzoin

Mix all the dry ingredients together. Blend or rub until very fine. Rub through a fine sieve. Mix the oils and tinctures together and drip into the mixed powders, stirring constantly to avoid lumping. Store in a container with a very tight-fitting lid.

A relaxing foot bath ready for tired feet

DOUCHES

I feel that douches are only warranted to help cure a local infection in the vagina. Regular douching can interfere with the acid/alkali balance and the natural and necessary secretions.

The only time that vaginal secretions smell unpleasant is when there is infection present or if regular washing is neglected.

If you are douching to cure a local infection you should persist, three times a day, for one week only. If the infection hasn't shown a marked improvement in this time you will need to find professional help to diagnose the problem. Undiagnosed, untreated vaginal discharge can lead to, or be indicative of, serious problems.

INGREDIENTS FOR DOUCHING

Bicarbonate of soda	Mugwort
Cider vinegar	Myrrh
Comfrey	Peppermint
Lavender	Rosemary
Marjoram	Tea tree
Mint	Yarrow

HERBAL DOUCHE

1 Prepare an infusion or decoction using herbs from the list above. Prepare fresh each time or store, covered, in the refrigerator for no longer than 24 hours.
2 Cool (or heat) to lukewarm. Pour into the container of a douche bag (bags can be obtained from pharmacies).
3 Sit, leaning back, on the toilet and insert the nozzle of the douche into the vagina. Allow the liquid to bathe the inside of the vagina (the liquid will run out but it's not necessary for it to stay inside).

THRUSH

Thrush is probably the most common vaginal problem experienced by women. It's uncomfortable, itchy and often occurs when other complaints such as cystitis are present (or it can cause cystitis), all of which is debilitating, tiring and demoralising.

Here are a few tips which should help to both prevent and cure thrush:
➤ If you are taking antibiotics eat at least 3 cups (600g/20oz) of live acidophilus yoghurt daily (buy a good quality acidophilus yoghurt).
➤ Use the yoghurt as a douche and/or dip a tampon in the yoghurt and insert into the vagina. Add 2 drops tincture of myrrh, 2 drops lavender oil and 4 drops tea tree oil to each 50ml ($1\frac{2}{3}$fl oz) of yoghurt. Change every 2 hours.
➤ Douche (instructions above) with 1 teaspoon tincture of myrrh in 1 cup (250ml/8fl oz) of warm water. Wash the area twice a day using the same mixture, freshly prepared. Dry with soft toilet paper and dispose of the paper down the toilet. Thrush is catching, so partners should treat themselves. (It's thought that men are 'symptomless' carriers of the infection.)
➤ Dissolve 2 tablespoons bicarbonate of soda or $\frac{1}{2}$ cup (125ml/4fl oz) Vinegar of the Four Thieves (see Skin Tonics) in 2 litres ($3\frac{1}{2}$ pints) of warm water in a bowl which is big enough to put your bottom in (this is known as a 'sitz bath'). Sit in the bowl, hold the vagina as open as you can and try to 'swoosh' some of the mixture inside. This 'bottom bath' often cures the thrush and certainly relieves the burning.
➤ Don't wear synthetic knickers, tights or pantihose, tight jeans or any tight clothing.
➤ Take a B complex vitamin capsule, garlic capsules and acidophilus capsules daily.
➤ Cut spices, alcohol and sugar entirely out except for natural sugars found in fruits and vegetables.

LEUCORRHOEA

This is a thick, white discharge which is non-infectious. Use the sitz bath or douche.

ACNE AND BLACKHEADS

Acne is a distressing and disfiguring complaint and is mainly a teenage problem but can occur in older people as well. Women who have a tendency to acne are most likely to have an outbreak during menopause and also during pre-menstruation.

As with most skin problems, acne treatment begins within the body; external treatments can only ever be a temporary solution. In order to get the best treatment for this condition it's wise to seek help from a professional. Naturopaths or homeopaths will take a careful history to determine the main cause and will devise a comprehensive course of treatment.

If you use the following programme for three to four weeks you will see a marked difference in your skin, body, emotions and mind.

➤ Make sure your bowels are functioning well.
➤ Eat lots of raw and cooked vegetables every day.
➤ Make a positive and conscious decision to cut out or down on junk food.
➤ Take a multivitamin capsule plus extra vitamins—B_6, E and C, and 15mg of zinc, and evening primrose capsules daily.
➤ Have some exercise every day. This will stimulate the circulation, lymphatic system, bladder and bowels and allow them to perform their toxin-removing functions. Increased circulation also brings healing nutrients and oxygen to the skin in increased quantities.
➤ Drink six to eight glasses of filtered water a day (tea, coffee, juices and others don't count).
➤ Treat your face to ten minutes of sunlight every day, preferably early morning or late afternoon.
➤ Drastically reduce salt intake (this has resulted in partial or complete cure for some people).
➤ Before breakfast, drink a glass of filtered water into which you have squeezed the juice of a lemon with no sweetener. The first morning is awful and then you start to look forward to it!
➤ Talk to a doctor about Retin A therapy.
➤ Lastly—relax. Join a stress management or meditation group; budget time for fun.

Externally there is quite a lot you can do to help reduce inflammation and promote healing:

➤ Wash the face three times a day using very mild soap which contains glycerine, then rinse well with lukewarm water—never use hot or cold water. Splash with the Herbal Rinse Lotion.
➤ Try to avoid using make-up or cover make-up. I know that this is hard but you stand a better chance of healing if you do this. Use only the Herbal Healing Oil and Herbal Night Oil on your skin. The powerful essences will kill bacteria, reduce inflammation and promote healing. Leave for five to ten minutes and blot the face with a tissue to remove the surplus.
➤ Have a facial steam once or twice a week using the Cleansing Steam Oils for Acne (see Aromatherapy and Perfumes).
➤ Never be tempted to squeeze a pimple.

BLACKHEADS

When the sebaceous glands oversecrete and the excess sebum doesn't move out of the duct, a blackhead results. The safest way to remove blackheads is to steam the skin, using boiling water and a few drops of antiseptic oil.

BLACKHEAD STEAM

1 Three-quarters fill a bowl with boiling water.
2 Put 1 drop tea tree oil and 2 drops geranium oil on the water.
3 Cover your head with a towel forming a closed tent around the bowl and your head.
4 Steam for about 10 minutes keeping your face about 30cm (12in) away from the water.
5 Pat the skin dry and, with cotton wool wrapped round your nails, gently press the skin on either side of the blackhead until it pops out.
6 Splash the skin with the following mixture:

2 tablespoons purified water
2 teaspoons distilled witch hazel
1 drop geranium oil
2 drops cypress oil

Mix all ingredients together. Splash on the skin.

DEODORANTS

Fresh perspiration has little odour but as it decomposes it develops mild to 'yuck' smells. The strength of perspiration odour seems to be determined by many factors—puberty or other hormonal changes, high intake of meat, 'junk' foods or alcohol and stress.

Synthetic clothing doesn't allow perspiration to evaporate and this compounds the problem. There is a condition called 'hyperhydrosis' in which the perspiration from the underarms is excessive and also can smell very unpleasant. This condition needs to be attended to by a professional as it may require surgery (the excision of the sweat glands towards the back of the armpits).

The following deodorants aren't as strong as the commercial varieties but are very nice to use and don't contain any dubious ingredients.

Deodorant Powder

½ teacup unperfumed talcum powder
½ teacup arrowroot powder
½ teaspoon ground cloves
1 tablespoon ground coriander seed
1 tablespoon dried and powdered sage leaves
1 tablespoon dried and powdered lavender flowers
1 tablespoon dried and powdered rosemary leaves
20 drops lavender oil
20 drops clary sage
10 drops rosemary oil
10 drops patchouli oil

Sieve the powders, herbs and spices together into a large bowl. Add the oils, a drop at a time, to the dry ingredients. Stir constantly to prevent lumping. Store the mixture in airtight containers.

Unperfumed Foot and Underarm Deodorant Powder

1 teacup unperfumed talcum powder
1 teacup arrowroot powder
2 teaspoons bicarbonate of soda

Mix all the ingredients together in a bowl or jar.

Quickie Deodorant

Use distilled witch hazel as an underarm splash.

Deodorant Lotion

90ml (3fl oz) distilled witch hazel
1 teaspoon glycerine
30 drops clary sage oil
10 drops lavender oil
10 drops thyme oil
10 drops patchouli oil
5 drops sandalwood oil

Blend all the ingredients in a 125ml (4fl oz) bottle. Shake well to mix and leave for 4 days before using. Shake before use.

Floral Deodorant Splash

This is an excellent deodorant splash which works well on most people.

60ml (2fl oz) white vinegar
30ml (1fl oz) distilled witch hazel
30ml (1fl oz) triple strength willow bark and orange peel decoction
5 drops thyme oil
5 drops lavender oil
10 drops orange oil
5 drops sandalwood oil

Mix all the ingredients in a 125ml (4fl oz) bottle. Shake well to mix and leave for 4 days before using. Shake before use.

Bath tray from Line and Lace of Balmain

Deodorant Powder in the making, a beautiful alternative to commercial varieties

MOTHERS
AND BABIES

There can be no more satisfying time in a woman's life than the nine months of pregnancy. This is a time for looking inwards to commune with the unborn but very aware human being growing within.

It's often said and is usually true that a woman is at her most beautiful during pregnancy. The extra hormones seem to give glossy, strong hair and a clear, blooming complexion. The early hormonal changes can however result in facial spots and greasy hair. It's usual for these depressing changes to settle down after the first four months so if you are experiencing them, hang in there—all will pass with the morning sickness. (The old trick of eating two plain arrowroot biscuits before lifting your head off the pillow in the morning usually fixes the morning sickness.) Gentle swimming and cycling are important to keep your body strong and supple.

The quality and variety of the food eaten is of paramount importance. The baby will always take the nutrition it needs and any deficiencies will be experienced by the mother.

Remember that anything experienced by you will also be experienced by your baby whether it is food, drink, inhaled fumes or chemicals, music, anger, unhappiness or joy. Try to surround yourself with beautiful things and cultivate tranquillity during the waiting months so that your baby will be born peaceful and contented.

The recipes in this section are for external use only, as specific advice should be obtained before taking internal remedies when pregnant.

OILS

As soon as pregnancy is confirmed it's time to start taking extra care of the skin on the tummy, thighs, bottom and breasts. Stretch marks can be avoided but not cured. Essential oils pass through the skin and are experienced by your baby so don't increase or change the recommended oils.

Commercial baby oil is usually mineral oil and not good to use on anyone—certainly not on new and tender skin. The best fixed oils for baby are virgin olive oil and almond oil. These should be used alone for the first couple of days as most essential oils are too powerful to use on newborn babies and there are very few which are safe to use until the baby is at least two to three months old.

It's safer to make a Herb Oil Base using the special baby herbs, German and Roman chamomile and lavender. Chamomile and lavender oil may be used for babies after the first forty-eight hours but the amount must never exceed 10 drops total essential oils in 100ml (3$\frac{1}{3}$fl oz) carrier oil. This herb oil may be used for general skin care, to remove cradle cap, and as the oil in the 'bottom cream' recipes following.

TTBB Oil

(You have to guess what TTBB means!)

150ml (5fl oz) triple strength herb oil made from calendula, comfrey root and nettle
3 teaspoons almond oil
3 teaspoons carrot oil
2 teaspoons avocado oil
1 teaspoon wheat germ oil
2 x 250 IU vitamin E capsules
20 drops mandarin oil
20 drops lavender oil
1 tablespoon vodka

Mix all the ingredients in a 200ml (6$\frac{1}{2}$fl oz) bottle. Shake the bottle well before use.

Massage the oil thoroughly into the skin of the breasts and from the waist down to the knees (bottom too—bottoms can get stretch marks!)

Almond Wash for Sensitive Skins

Almond milk is a lovely wash for babies' sensitive skins. It can be used over the entire body and can be stored for 3 days in the refrigerator.

Blend 40 almonds to a pulp with 2 cups (500ml/16fl oz) of boiling water. Stand until lukewarm. Strain through cheesecloth (muslin).

Teddy bear from Linen and Lace of Balmain

Nipple Cream

Use from early pregnancy and wash away the cream before feeding your baby.

PHASE A

2 tablespoons lanolin

3 teaspoons honey

2 tablespoons triple strength calendula oil (see Making a Herb Oil Base in Chapter One)

PHASE B

2 tablespoons purified water

PHASE C

20 drops evening primrose oil

30 drops tincture of benzoin

Melt the phase A ingredients gently in a double boiler, stirring often until the mixture is liquid but not overheated.

Add the phase B ingredient and stir well to incorporate. Add the phase C ingredients when the mixture is 50°C (120°F) or just below. Stir well until no water or oil droplets can be seen. Pot in sterilised containers and cap immediately.

'Bottom Cream'

PHASE A

1 cube (15g/½oz) beeswax

60g (2oz) lanolin

100ml (3⅓fl oz) Herb Oil Base (see Chapter One)

PHASE B

2 teaspoons calendula tincture

1 teaspoon tincture of benzoin

Melt the phase A ingredients gently in a double boiler stirring often until the mixture is liquid but not overheated.

Add the phase B ingredients, stirring well to incorporate and until no water or oil droplets can be seen. Pot in sterilised containers and cap immediately.

Vitamin A 'Bottom Cream'

Cod-liver oil doesn't smell too good but it's a terrific healer for bottoms which are raw and sore. Use a nappy-liner to protect the nappy.

PHASE A

1 tablespoon lanolin

1 cube (15g/½oz) beeswax

PHASE B

2 tablespoons olive oil

1 tablespoon cod-liver oil

2 teaspoons unperfumed talcum powder

Melt the phase A ingredients gently in a double boiler stirring often until the mixture is liquid but not overheated.

Heat the phase B oils slightly and mix well with the talcum powder. Add the phase B mixture to the phase A mixture and stir well to incorporate. Pot in sterilised containers and cap immediately.

FOR FRETFUL BABIES

If baby is very fretful try putting a few drops of lavender oil on a piece of cloth and hanging it in the baby's bedroom (not too close to the cot).

TALCUM POWDERS

Home-made baby powders have the advantage of containing only natural ingredients and are useful to keep the tender little creases in a baby's body dry and sweet, but too much powder can clog the tiny pores and cause problems—only the lightest dusting is needed. (For more information see Talcum Powder in the Glossary.)

In the following recipes, the finished mixture of ground herbs and powder must be sieved through the very finest sieve. Coarse particles would be irritating to the skin. I use an electric coffee grinder and pass the ground material through a sieve, regrind the particles remaining in the sieve and so on. I finish by regrinding the whole lot and passing it through a superfine sieve or rubbing it through cheesecloth. Make sure that the container in which you keep the powder is absolutely airtight or it will become lumpy.

Nappy Rash Powder

Baby Powder

A lovely, soothing and healing powder for your baby. It is a time-consuming recipe but it can be made in much larger quantities to last.

30g (1oz) dried chamomile leaves
30g (1oz) dried calendula petals
30g (1oz) rolled oats
30g (1oz) arrowroot powder
30g unperfumed talcum powder

Grind all the ingredients to a fine powder. Pass through a fine-grade sieve and then cheesecloth.

Nappy Rash Powder

Zinc oxide is for healing or preventing nappy rash. When combined with healing herbs, is the best ever powder to prevent or cure nappy rash.

1 teacup cornflour
1 teacup unperfumed talcum powder
2 tablespoons zinc oxide powder
2 tablespoons dried calendula petals powdered
2 tablespoons dried chamomile flowers powdered
20 drops chamomile oil

Finely sieve all the dry ingredients into a bowl. Add the oil a drop at a time, stirring constantly to prevent lumps forming.

CHAPTER THREE

HAIR CARE

Very few people seem satisfied with their hair. In the

pursuit of their dream of thick, glossy hair, many women

and men buy increasingly expensive and impressive-

sounding preparations. The money would be far better spent

in their own kitchens making real, honest-to-goodness

preparations which will really improve the condition and

appearance of the hair.

Hairbrushes and comb from Crabtree & Evelyn

*A good quality natural bristle
brush will last for years*

BETTER HAIR

It takes a little courage to change from commercial shampoos and conditioners to the home-made variety as we have been brain-washed into believing that the more we pay, the better the product must be. The fact is, manufacturers of skin and hair care products couldn't afford to make the high-quality products which we can make at home. They have to pay for machinery, labels, jars and bottles and spend millions of dollars on advertising. There has to be plenty of margin to pay representatives, middlemen, wholesalers and retailers!

Because of these costs, the contents have to be cheap and need to have a very long shelf life (they usually consist of large numbers of unpronounceable chemicals which never 'go off'). The customer is last in line when it comes to priorities. I have worked for some of the biggest multinational cosmetic companies and know how little the contents of the bottle are worth—usually a few cents. I have also owned a business that made skin and hair products, and I know how small a profit margin there is when you use expensive, wholesome, natural ingredients.

New labelling regulations make it a legal obligation that most product labels must display a list of contents. The list shows the contents in order of percentage, the highest being first, down to the smallest last. Take a look at the average herbal shampoo (or vitamin E cream, for instance) and you will usually find that the herb content is the last on the list. It's acceptable to call a product 'herbal' regardless of how small the herb content is.

In our kitchens we can use the best: cream; butter; honey; non-synthetic essential oils; cold-pressed oil and so on. Rest assured—your 'Maison Moi' skin and hair care range is going to be the finest in the world.

Many commercial shampoos have formulae very similar to carpet shampoos. The detergent is so strong and strips the hair to such an extent that a wax conditioner is needed to create manageable, artificially shiny hair—another sale! Most conditioners coat the hair with waxy substances which, over a period of time, create a build-up which results in weakened hair.

In my book *Herbcraft*, I make the following remarks:

'When I was a child we washed our hair with soap and rainwater; occasionally an egg would be massaged in to give body. The finishing touch was a herbal vinegar or lemon rinse. I have photographs of myself with strong, glossy brown hair (totally straight and not blonde, which was the great grief of my life) and I remember brushing my mother's hair, so black and shiny that it looked polished. Conditioners, permanent waves, hair colourants from a bottle and even 'bought' shampoos were rare and yet most people, unless they were sick, had a very good head of hair.'

There is a factor in hair strength and appearance which is rarely considered, and that is that the hair and nails are 'barometers' of health and are frequently the first part of our bodies to warn us that all is not well. Hair can become thin and lifeless; nails become brittle with ridges and white spots.

The external care which we lavish on our hair is going to be largely wasted if we don't get enough sleep, if we are stressed or if our nutrition is being neglected.

THE NATURE OF HAIR

Each hair on your head and body is 'dead'. It is made up of a protein substance called keratin, which is produced from a follicle in the dermis (see The Nature of Skin in Chapter Two). The hair is released from the follicle naturally (when brushing or washing), and the follicle then produces another hair. The process is accelerated by accidental loss, so hair that has been pulled out usually re-grows very quickly. The expression 'hair pulled out by the roots' is inaccurate as the follicle is the 'root' and this can't be pulled out.

The follicles produce and shed hairs independently of each other. If this were not so we would be bald for a while and then have an unmanageably thick head of hair for a while.

Everyone has approximately 100,000 hair follicles in their scalp but the thickness of the hair shaft may differ greatly depending on your genes. The follicles are fed from nutrients in the blood supply to the scalp. If nutrients are absent in the blood the very greedy follicles won't be able to grow healthy hair. This is a perfect example of good nutrition being an important factor.

Hair is composed of three layers. The centre is called the medulla, next is the cortex and the outer layer is the cuticle. This outer layer protects the other two and is formed of overlapping scales. If hair is treated harshly by overuse of sprays, too much sunlight or wind, excessive shampooing, harsh shampoos, overheating during drying, or overcolouring/bleaching/perming, the cuticle may dry out, crack and expose the vulnerable inner layers. The hair will then split, break or become unmanageable and dull.

Oil for the hair shaft is supplied from a gland which is situated in the dermis but is closer to the scalp than the follicle.

Research seems to show that hair cannot be 'fed' from the scalp. It can only receive nutrients through the blood supply to the follicle. We can however protect and improve the appearance of our hair by using natural ingredients.

HAIR TYPES

There are many different types of hair, all of which are inherited. You won't be able to change your hair type but there are several ways of getting the best from the type with which nature or your parents blessed you.

FINE HAIR

Fine hair lacks body and tends to be limp but this type of hair can look and feel lovely if treated with both pre-shampoo and after-shampoo conditioners which give 'body' to the silky strands.

If you have fine hair you need to be gentle with it. Use a soft bristle brush with rounded ends on the bristles. Don't expose it to too much sun or wind. Don't overcolour, perm or bleach as this hair type becomes brittle and breaks easily.

Avoid regular use of hair rollers or wearing your hair in tightly pulled-back styles such as 'pony tails' as this will stress the delicate structure of the hair.

COARSE HAIR

Coarse hair is thick, strong and wiry. If this is your hair type, be happy! You are very lucky as coarse hair will resist a lot of abuse without splitting or breaking. It's not always necessary to condition coarse hair but if there is not as much shine as you would like, an after-shampoo conditioner and between-shampoo hair dressing would be beneficial.

THIN HAIR

Very often fine as well. This type of hair needs plenty of pre- and after-shampoo conditioners which contain protein, such as egg and milk, to give an appearance of fullness. Treat the hair gently, never use harsh treatments and avoid overcolouring or perming. Choose a soft brush with rounded bristles and don't overdo the brushing—thirty to forty strokes are ample.

OILY HAIR

Overactive sebaceous glands are responsible for the excessive oil which plagues people with this type of hair. Shampooing every day can aggravate the problem as the glands become even more active with the constant stimulation. Dry shampoos are an excellent compromise as they remove the grease effectively between shampoos. Don't use very hot water when shampooing, and brush the hair gently the whole length of the shaft to distribute the oil.

Oily hair benefits from the use of vinegar or lemon rinses as these close the hair cuticles, strip the excessive oil and leave the hair shining and manageable.

DRY HAIR

Any type of hair may have a problem with dryness. Dry hair is usually dull, has a tendency to breaking and is difficult to style. The management of this type of hair depends on not aggravating the situation by using harsh shampoos, hot dryers or curling wands; exposing the hair to too much sun and/or wind; neglecting to rinse and shampoo after swimming; too vigorous brushing; and insufficient moisturising/conditioning.

HINTS FOR HEALTHY HAIR

So...where do we begin in this search for naturally healthy hair?

➤ Check the discussion on nutrients in the diet at the end of this list to make sure that you are getting optimum nutrition. Healthy hair comes from within. Don't expect an overnight change, as hair might take weeks to show the benefits.

➤ Unless your hair is really dirty, it only needs washing once a week. Frequent washing stimulates the oil glands which makes oily hair conditions worse. Try a dry shampoo if you can't bear to wait a week.

➤ Shampooing once is enough. Shampooing twice will strip every trace of natural oil from the hair; leaving it completely unmanageable. Clean hair shouldn't be 'squeaky'—if it is it means that there is no trace of natural oil left, and it's this natural oil which gives shine.

➤ Avoid commercial shampoos or at least buy the most natural one you can find in the health food shop. Even these shampoos can be improved and made to last longer by the addition of concentrated herb infusions.

➤ Buy a pure bristle hairbrush and check by tapping against your palm to make sure that the ends of the bristles are rounded, not sharp. Good brushes are expensive but if cared for will last for years and years. Bend over when brushing your hair and be gentle—thirty to forty strokes are plenty. Start brushing at the scalp and bring the brush through to the end of the hair; this distributes the oil evenly. Bending over also brings the blood to the scalp which is beneficial to the hair follicle.

➤ Buy a wide-toothed comb. Teeth which are too close together can pull out a lot of hair.

➤ If your hair is pulled back in pony tails, plaits, hair rollers or any hairstyle which causes tension for extended periods of time, you could develop a condition called traction alopecia. This means that you are losing hair because you are pulling it out!

- Overuse of chemicals to colour hair and using heat to dry your hair could result in brittle hair which breaks. If you don't do either of these and your hair is still brittle, look to your diet.
- Chlorinated water or sea water can damage hair. Rinse the hair immediately after swimming, and shampoo as soon as possible using a good conditioning and moisturising treatment before and after the shampoo.
- Massage the scalp regularly to increase the flow of blood to the roots of the hair. To massage the scalp you place all the fingers and thumbs firmly on the scalp and move the scalp itself. Don't rub—rubbing would result in the hair being pulled out, which rather defeats the object of the massage.
- Ensure healthy hair by including the following in your diet:
- Essential fatty acids, to condition and lubricate
- Iron, as its absence makes hair dull and brittle
- Sulphur, needed to maintain hair colour
- Copper, as lack of this mineral damages hair
- Zinc, the same as copper
- Vitamin B complex, as lack of these vitamins causes dullness, scaling, dandruff, greyness and balding
- Vitamin C, to maintain capillaries which carry blood to the follicles

GREY HAIR

Grey hair is a mixture of your natural colour and white hairs. Hair colour is decided by the melanin structure and by genetics. Greyness is caused by lessening of melanin production; if your mother or father went grey when young, the chances are that you might also.

HAIR LOSS

The following drugs can cause mild to serious hair loss: two or more aspirin a day; birth control pills (see your doctor regarding a change if you notice hair falling out); diet pills; cortisone (which can make hair grow on your face and fall out of your head); anticoagulants and amphetamines; chemotherapy. Major shock such as a serious accident, or stress such as prolonged illness, divorce, death of someone close, or liver disease caused by years of heavy drinking, can all cause hair loss. If the situation is remedied and the stress brought under control, the hair loss is not usually permanent and the hair follicles will usually begin to grow hair again within weeks or months.

If you are a woman who suffers from very heavy periods and you are losing hair, it could be a sign that you are iron deficient. A blood test would be indicated in this case. See also the list of iron-rich foods in Chapter Seven.

Hypo/hyperthyroidism are other conditions which may cause hair loss and where a blood test is necessary. Hair loss is natural in the spring and autumn as we (being animals!) moult naturally during these seasons. Don't panic as this is a perfectly natural phenomenon.

If you are a new mother you have a lot to contend with: dirty nappies, a windy baby, broken nights and now—to cap it all (bad pun) your hair starts to fall out. Don't worry—it will grow again as the body recovers from the birth and adjusts to the new demands being made on it. If you fret about it you will lose more. Make sure that you take a nap when the baby is asleep—the dishes and vacuuming will wait until your partner gets home!

INGREDIENTS
FOR HAIR CARE

DRY HAIR

Carrot
Egg yolk
Full cream milk
Geranium
Glycerine
Honey
Lavender
Parsley
Rosemary

DAMAGED HAIR

Calendula
Carrot
Chamomile
Clary sage
Egg yolk
Full cream milk
Glycerine
Honey
Lavender
Sandalwood
Thyme

MOISTURISING

Carrot
Geranium
Jojoba
Lemon
Rosemary
Thyme

OILY HAIR

Basil
Eucalyptus
Honey
Lavender
Lemon
Peppermint
Rosemary
Skim milk
Whole egg
Willow bark
Witch hazel
Yarrow

DANDRUFF

Basil
Carrot
Cypress
Lavender
Mint
Nettle
Parsley
Rosemary

REDUCING HAIR LOSS

Carrot
Chamomile
Clary sage
Cypress
Lemon
Sage

HAIR CONDITIONERS

Almond oil
Basil oil
Castor oil
Coconut oil
Egg yolk
Glycerine
Honey
Jojoba oil
Lavender oil
Lavender infusion
Mayonnaise
Nettle leaf infusion
Olive oil
Rosemary oil
Rosemary infusion
Sage leaf infusion
Southernwood leaf infusion

COLOURANTS

BLONDE

Calendula petals
Chamomile
Lemon juice, diluted
Purple loosestrife, dried leaves,
shoots
Turmeric
Rhubarb root

BROWN

Espresso coffee
Sage
Strong black tea
Walnut

DANDRUFF RINSES

Chamomile triple strength
infusion
Cider vinegar
Lemon grass triple strength
infusion
Lemon juice rinse
Nettle triple strength infusion
Parsley triple strength infusion
Rosemary triple strength
infusion
Willow bark triple strength
infusion

DARK HAIR

Cider vinegar
Nettle triple strength infusion
Parsley triple strength infusion
Rosemary triple strength
infusion
Sage triple strength infusion
Southernwood triple strength
infusion

RED

Henna
Red hibiscus

TO COVER GREY

Black tea
Elderberries (for blue tone)
Green orange peel
Sage
Strong espresso coffee
Walnut inner husks

FAIR HAIR

Chamomile double strength
infusion
Calendula double strength
infusion
Elderflower triple strength
infusion
Lemon juice, diluted
White willow bark decoction

DRY SHAMPOOS

Cornmeal
Oats, ground
Orris root powder

BLACK

Henna-reng
Jacob's ladder
St John's wort

HAIR TREATMENTS

The pH of hair is slightly acidic in the same way as skin, but there is no such thing as an acidic shampoo because alkalinity is needed to degrease hair. Soaps and shampoos are alkaline by nature, which enables them to do a good cleaning job but which also causes the overlapping scales on the hair shaft to open and separate. The hair then has a tendency to lawlessness, standing away from the scalp and having a lacklustre, flyaway appearance.

It's important that rinses and conditioners are mildly acidic to counteract the alkalinity of the shampoo and to cause the overlapping scales on the hair shaft to close and lie flat and overlap once more. When this happens the hair has a shiny smooth appearance and the inside of the hair shaft is protected.

Most commercial conditioners are a wax formula which creates a build-up of wax on the hair shaft. This slowly but surely weakens the hair (this build-up will take about 3–4 weeks to dissolve so don't expect immediate miracles from your change of treatment). Natural conditioners coat the hair shaft with protein provided by gelatine, egg yolk or milk—these give body and shine, prevent static build-up and so give manageability. The following recipes are for natural pre-shampoo treatments, shampoos, rinses and conditioners. They may take a little getting used to but will reward you with the best head of hair ever to crown you.

PRE-SHAMPOO TREATMENTS

Simply Egg
ALL HAIR TYPES

2 eggs

Beat the eggs in a small bowl until frothy. Massage gently into the hair. Cover hair with a plastic shower cap or a towel wrung out in hot water. Leave for 20 minutes. Shampoo with a mild herbal shampoo.

Milk and Honey
DRY/DAMAGED/FINE HAIR

1 egg yolk, beaten
1 teaspoon runny honey
1 tablespoon fresh milk
4 drops rosemary or lavender oil
dried milk powder to mix

Combine the egg yolk, honey, milk and lavender oil in a bowl. Add enough milk powder to make a paste. Massage gently into the hair. Cover the hair with a plastic shower cap or a towel wrung out in very hot water. Leave for 20 minutes. Shampoo with a mild herbal shampoo.

Mayonnaise
ALL EXCEPT VERY OILY HAIR

1 egg yolk
1 tablespoon cider vinegar
1 tablespoon castor oil
1 tablespoon olive oil, approximately

Beat the egg and vinegar together with a whisk or in a blender. Add the oils in a thin stream while beating until the mixture is thick. You may need to add more olive oil if the mixture is too thick. Massage gently into the hair. Cover the hair with a plastic shower cap or a towel wrung out in very hot water. Leave for 20 minutes. Shampoo with a mild herbal shampoo.

Citrus Egg
OILY HAIR

1 egg, beaten
1 teaspoon runny honey
1 teaspoon lemon juice
1 tablespoon water
3 drops lemon oil
dried milk powder

Combine the egg, honey, juice, water and oil in a bowl. Add enough milk powder to make a smooth paste. Massage gently into the hair. Cover the hair with a plastic shower cap or a towel wrung out in very hot water. Leave for 20 minutes. Shampoo with a mild herbal shampoo.

A selection of hair treatments

Candles from Crabtree & Evelyn; flowers by Lisa Milasas

Hot oil

ALL HAIR TYPES EXCEPT OILY

This simple treatment works particularly well on very dry, damaged hair and is also a good treatment for dandruff as it loosens the scaly dried sebum from the scalp. Heat a mixture of olive, coconut and castor oil to lukewarm. Massage gently into the hair. Cover the head with a piece of towelling wrung out in very hot water and a plastic shower cap. Wrap the head in a hot towel. Change the towel when it cools. Repeat a few times and don't shampoo for at least an hour. Follow with a herbal shampoo.

SHAMPOOS

Herbal Oil Shampoo Base

This shampoo contains essential oils and won't 'go off' in the same way as those using fresh herbal infusions. By using the table of Ingredients for Hair Care, you can choose essential oils suitable for your hair type. It's fine to include egg or any other shampoo enricher but don't add these until you are ready to use it.

By making up a quantity of the shampoo base each member of the family will be able to devise his or her own tailor-made shampoo.

100g (3⅓oz) soap flakes (e.g. Lux) or finely
grated soap
4 cups (1 litre/32fl oz) purified water or
rainwater, heated
2 teaspoons borax

Mix all the ingredients in a bowl until dissolved. Cool and pour into a large jar. Mix well before using. Mix a total of 100 drops of your chosen essential oils with 1 cup (250ml/8fl oz) of the basic mixture. Blend really well. The mixture may go lumpy on standing—this doesn't matter, just give it a good stir until blended. This amount will provide enough for several shampoos.

Protein Shampoo

DAMAGED/DRY/FINE HAIR

1 cup (250ml/8fl oz) triple strength
rosemary/lavender infusion
1 tablespoon powdered gelatine
1 teaspoon lanolin
1 cup (250ml/8fl oz) baby shampoo

Heat the infusion until almost boiling. Sprinkle over the gelatine and stir until dissolved. Add the lanolin and stir until well mixed. Add the shampoo and stir until well mixed. Bottle.

Mix together 1 beaten egg and 1 tablespoon of the prepared shampoo. Massage into wet hair, leave for 4–5 minutes, massaging gently. Rinse very well in lukewarm water.

Castile and Herb Shampoo

ALL HAIR TYPES

This shampoo is gentle and very sweet smelling. Choose the herbs from the table on Ingredients for Hair Care (include one or two aromatics). Use an acidic rinse following the shampoo. If you want to use your home-made castile soap (see Chapter Five) for this recipe you should grate the soap and dissolve it in some warm water to reduce it to a thin jelly consistency before adding it to the herbal infusion.

2 tablespoons finely chopped fresh herbs
1 cup (250ml/8fl oz) purified or rainwater
¾ cup (185ml/6fl oz) liquid castile soap

Add the herbs to the water in a saucepan, simmer covered for 30 minutes. Stand for 1 hour. Strain. Simmer, covered, until reduced to ¼ cup (60ml/2fl oz). Cool. Add the castile soap, mix and bottle.

Health Food Store Shampoo

ALL HAIR TYPES

For those of you who have very little time to make your own shampoo, here is a very acceptable compromise—this recipe will save money as well as extending the shampoo. The resultant shampoo will be thinner than usual but does a really good job. You will need a bottle of baby shampoo or the best herbal shampoo you can find, plus an empty shampoo bottle. Divide the shampoo between the two bottles.

Choose the herbs from the table on Ingredients for Hair Care and chop finely before adding to the water. If you have dry hair you can melt a teaspoonful of lanolin into the hot herbal infusion. Mix really well before adding the shampoo.

1 teacup finely chopped fresh herbs
purified water or rainwater to cover

Simmer the herbs and water in a covered saucepan for 30 minutes. Stand 1 hour. Strain. Divide between the two bottles of shampoo.

Conditioning Shampoo

This shampoo cleans and conditions in one operation.

1 teaspoon powdered gelatine
2 tablespoons hot water
1 egg, beaten
1 teaspoon runny honey
1 drop lavender oil
2 drops rosemary oil
1 tablespoon shampoo

Sprinkle the gelatine over the water and stir until dissolved. Cool. Add the egg, honey and oils, mix well. Add the shampoo and mix well. Massage into wet hair and leave on while bathing or showering. Rinse well with lukewarm water.

Lentil Shampoo

ALL HAIR TYPES

On one of my visits to India I became friendly with a very poor Indian woman and her family. They were the ultimate recyclers, existing mainly on things thrown away by Westerners. I didn't speak her language and she didn't speak English but we managed to communicate very well.

They lived in a burned-out bus which had no floor but sat uncompromisingly on the earth. In one corner was a pile of rags which served as a bed for husband, wife and four children. In another corner was a wok and a flat iron pan with which they cooked their simple diet of rice, lentils and chappatis. These few things were their entire belongings as the only clothes they owned were on their backs.

On one of my visits to the bus I found my friend rubbing a paste of mashed cooked lentils into her hair. She offered a small handful to me and even though I was bewildered, I took the pulp and massaged it into my hair and scalp. We then went outside and poured water from the well (alive with amoebas and other unmentionables) over each other's head, then sat in the sun near a jasmine vine to dry our hair and talk in sign language about life and love.

That's it! This whole story was just to share with you this extraordinary shampoo which leaves hair clean, soft and shiny. No need for anything except cooked, mashed lentils and rinsing water, and (desirable but not essential) a good friend with whom to share the experience.

Soapwort Shampoo
ALL HAIR TYPES

Soapwort (*saponaria officinalis*) has been used to clean and restore old and very fragile tapestries and silk hangings. If you are fortunate enough to have a lot of this herb growing in the garden you can utilise its gentle cleansing power by making it into shampoo.

Soapwort does its job without a lot of fuss. Since the advent of detergents we have become accustomed to lots of froth and bubble, but this really isn't necessary. We have been led to believe the fallacy that lots of froth means very clean clothes/hair/bodies.

If you live in a hard-water area you will need to add borax to the shampoo. The borax acts as a very mild preservative but this shampoo needs to be refrigerated and will only keep for about 2 weeks. Rainwater is ideal for washing anything as it is so soft.

Make a triple strength decoction using 2 good handfuls of finely chopped soapwort root, stems and leaves and 1 handful of your other chosen herbs. (Choose herbs suitable for your hair type from the table on Ingredients for Hair Care.) Leave to stand 24 hours before straining.

Add 1 teaspoon borax to 1 cup (250ml/8fl oz) warm decoction, dissolve and mix all together. Add 5 drops of essential oil (optional) before bottling. Shake well before use.

RINSES

Castile shampoos need to be followed by an acidic rinse to make hair manageable and to neutralise the alkalinity of the soap. Herb rinses are undoubtedly the nicest but 1 tablespoon vinegar or lemon juice in 1 cup (250ml/8fl oz) water is fine if you're short of time. Choose the herbs from the table on Ingredients for Hair Care. They can be the same as the ones used in the shampoo.

Herbal Hair Rinse

Make 4 cups (1 litre/32fl oz) of a triple strength infusion/decoction. Strain into a jug and cool to a usable heat. Add 1 tablespoon lemon juice, cider vinegar or Herb Vinegar (see Chapter One).

Place a bowl in the washbasin and pour the rinse over your hair, catching the surplus in the bowl. Empty the rinse back into the jug and repeat as long as you like (or until your arms go on strike!).

Quickie Rinse

Stale beer hair rinse. It's an oldie but it's a goodie. It's been around for years and is hard to beat. The more natural the beer the better. Don't worry—you won't smell like a 'pub bar the morning after'—the smell vanishes really quickly and your hair is left shiny and full of body.

Lavender Hair Rinse

Lavender is suitable for all hair types and the smell is so sweet and familiar that this vinegar rinse will be enjoyed by the whole family.

Make a Herb Vinegar (see Chapter One) using finely chopped lavender flowers. Strain. Repeat the process using more lavender flowers. Repeat a third time if you want a triple strength vinegar with a strong perfume. If you are feeling particularly rich and extravagant you can use half and half white wine vinegar and vodka instead of cider vinegar. Add ½ cup (125ml/4fl oz) to 4 cups (1 litre/32fl oz) warm water as a final rinse.

Rinsing with the beautifully fragrant Lavender Hair Rinse

CONDITIONERS

The following conditioners don't put layers of silicone on the hair shaft—they leave hair full-bodied, soft and glossy.

Honey Conditioner

ALL HAIR TYPES

1 beaten egg
1 teaspoon runny honey
1 teaspoon herbal/cider vinegar
dried skim milk powder

Combine the egg, honey and vinegar in a bowl. Add enough milk powder to make a smooth paste. Massage into the hair after shampooing, leave on the hair for a few minutes, then rinse lightly with lukewarm water.

Lavender and Basil Conditioner

ALL HAIR TYPES EXCEPT OILY

1 egg, beaten
1 teaspoon glycerine
2 drops light sesame oil
2 drops lavender oil
2 drops basil oil
dried skim milk powder

Beat the egg, glycerine and oils in a bowl. Add enough milk powder to make a smooth paste. Massage into the hair after shampooing, leave on the hair for a few minutes, then rinse lightly with lukewarm water.

Witch Hazel and Citrus Conditioner

OILY HAIR

2 tablespoons witch hazel
1 teaspoon runny honey
1 egg, beaten
2 drops lemon oil
dried skim milk powder

Combine the witch hazel, honey, egg and oil in a bowl. Add enough milk powder to make a smooth paste. Massage into the hair after shampooing, leave on the hair for a few minutes, then rinse lightly with lukewarm water.

SETTING LOTIONS

Any of the mucilages in Chapter One can be used as a setting lotion. Make a thinner mix than specified and use one of the 'hair herb' infusions instead of water to mix. When cool, a few drops of rosemary and lavender oil can be mixed in. Comb the thin gel through the hair before setting.

Quickie Setting Lotion 1

FOR FAIR OR OILY HAIR

1 tablespoon lemon juice
2–3 tablespoons water

Combine the juice and water in a spray bottle. Spray on the hair after washing. This lotion will discourage oil and will act like a natural hair lacquer to hold a set in place.

Quickie Setting Lotion 2

milk

water

Combine the milk and water using equal amounts of each. This makes a good setting lotion. Use skim milk for oily hair, full cream for all other hair types.

Gelatine Hair Set

MOST HAIR TYPES

This hair set gives body to fine, limp hair and helps all hair types to achieve a good set. Mix in a jug and pour over your head several times as a final rinse.

1 tablespoon gelatine
2 cups (500ml/16fl oz) very hot water
4 drops rosemary oil

Sprinkle the gelatine over the hot water and stir until the gelatine is dissolved. Cool to a usable temperature. Mix the oil in really well.

Setting Lotion

It's difficult to give precise amounts of ingredients for this recipe as the strength depends very much on individual preference. Try the quantities given below and adapt to suit yourself.

1 teaspoon gum tragacanth or pectin
1 tablespoon vodka
80–180ml ($2\frac{2}{3}$–6fl oz) water
$\frac{1}{2}$ teaspoon glycerine
4 drops rosemary oil
2 drops lavender oil

Mix the tragacanth and vodka and leave to swell. Mix in all the remaining ingredients and leave to thicken, stirring often. Bottle. Comb through the hair before setting or dilute with water and use as a final rinse.

Brush, comb and soap dish from Crabtree & Evelyn

*Setting lotions from natural
ingredients hold a set in place*

NATURAL COLOURANTS

Colouring hair with natural ingredients requires perseverance and care but the results are not only improved colour but healthier, shinier and fuller hair. Many books suggest using the herbs as a rinse but it has been my experience that the infusion/decoction needs to be left on the hair for some time to make an appreciable difference.

Henna (*Lawsonia inermis*) is a plant which yields a semi-permanent red dye from its dried leaves. It has been used in India and the Middle East for centuries to dye hair (and various parts of the body such as the palms of the hands and the soles of the feet).

Natural Hair Colourant: General Directions

The infusion in this recipe can be made in any quantity and frozen. It's very time-consuming to make a fresh batch each time. It will take a few treatments before an appreciable difference is noticed, but persevere and you will be rewarded!

Make a triple strength decoction, adding a teaspoon of cider vinegar to the herbs and boiling water. Simmer until a very strong colour has been obtained—stand overnight if necessary. Strain.

Add a pinch of salt and a teaspoon of glycerine. Mix well. Mix to a cream with fuller's earth or kaolin (or henna if you have decided to use it).

Shampoo the hair and towel dry. Massage the colourant thoroughly into the hair. Hold the head over a washbasin containing very hot water and steam for about 10 minutes. Cover the head with a plastic shower cap and leave for ½–1 hour or even longer if possible.

Work up colourant with a little warm water (don't shampoo), then rinse off thoroughly with lukewarm water.

NOTE: Henna may be mixed, in small quantities, to enrich the dyes obtained from other herbs and to make their colour last longer (herbal extracts used alone are rarely permanent). I can't tell you how much to use. Henna, like all natural products, varies in strength depending on the area in which it was grown and other variants, such as the type of hair and length of time the mixture is on the hair, will be factors in the finished effect.

Test the mixture on a small sample of hair before using it on the whole head. Remember that the effect will be strengthened by each successive application.

Mixing hair colourants

NATURAL HAIR COLOURANTS

PROPERTY	PLANT	PART USED	HOW TO USE
To colour hair red or to give red highlights to brown hair	Red hibiscus Henna	Petals	See the general directions in the recipe, this section. Follow the directions on the packet.

PROPERTY	PLANT	PART USED	HOW TO USE
To lighten blond hair and give honey highlights to mousy or faded blonde hair	Purple loosestrife Calendula Turmeric Chamomile	Dried leaves Petals Ground spice Flower heads	See the general directions in the recipe, this section. As above. As above. Dry, grind to powder, add equal quantities kaolin. Mix with water. Follow the general directions in the recipe, this section.
	Lemon	Juice	Dilute juice with equal amounts of water. Follow the general directions in the recipe, this section.

NATURAL HAIR COLOURANTS

PROPERTY	PLANT	PART USED	HOW TO USE
To add sheen and depth to faded black hair	Henna-reng		Follow the directions on the packet.
	Rosemary	Petals	See the general directions in the recipe, this section.
To cover grey hair or add blue tones	Sage	Leaves	See the general directions in the recipe, this section.
	Elder	Berries	As above.
	Walnut	Green outer underripe husk	As above.
	Black tea (acts as a fixative)	Leaves	As above.
	Espresso coffee		Use instead of the decoction in the recipe's general directions, this section.
To brighten and/or darken brown hair	Sage	Leaves	See the general directions in the recipe, this section.
	Alkanet	Root	As above.
	Walnut	Green outer underripe husk	As above.
	Black tea (acts as a fixative)	leaves	As above.
	Espresso coffee		Use instead of the decoction in the recipe's general directions, this section.

HAIR DRESSING

Hair dressings are applied to the hair between shampoos to keep the hair glossy and smooth. The best dressings are those which leave no greasy residue on the hair. See Chapter Six for recipes using essential oils which are absorbed into the hair shaft leaving the hair silky soft and sweet-smelling.

HAIR TONICS

Hair tonics are used for many reasons: to stimulate the flow of blood to the scalp and so encourage stronger hair growth; to relieve the irritation of dry, itchy and flaking scalp; as part of the treatment for dandruff; to reduce grease in oily hair; to moisturise dry hair. Choose the herbs for your hair tonic from the table on Ingredients for Hair Care. The recipe below is an example for you to follow, and is suitable for most hair types.

Herbal Hair Tonic
MOST HAIR TYPES

First make a triple strength decoction using as many as possible of the following herbs: nettle, comfrey root, rosemary, lavender, sage, southernwood, parsley, thyme and wormwood. Leave the herbs in the liquid for several hours before straining. This decoction freezes well and I usually make about 2 litres (3½ pints) and freeze it in small containers.

1 teaspoon borax
1 cup (250ml/8fl oz) hot triple strength decoction
20 drops rosemary oil
20 drops lavender oil
1 teaspoon rose-water
1 teaspoon cider vinegar

Dissolve the borax in the decoction, then allow it to cool. Add the oils, rose-water and vinegar, then bottle. Store tonic in the refrigerator. Shake well before use.

Sprinkle a little tonic onto the scalp. Using the pads of the fingers, massage the scalp by moving the skin firmly, not pulling at the roots of the hair. Finally brush the remaining tonic through the hair.

DANDRUFF TREATMENTS

There is no doubt that to suffer from dandruff is distressing. Those embarrassing little white flakes which cascade onto your shoulders to ruin the appearance of your immaculate ensemble don't do anything for your self-esteem. Dandruff is caused by excess sebum blocking the pore of the hair follicle and then drying out to little white flakes. It follows then that most dandruff sufferers have oily skin and hair.

If you have dandruff and you don't have oily hair, the problem may be stress. For reasons not yet understood, anxiety can cause dandruff.

Beware of 'dandruff shampoos'—the makers have an investment in keeping you hooked on their product forever—the shampoo keeps dandruff at bay, but doesn't cure the cause.

There are a few herbs which are especially valuable in the treatment of dandruff, and cider vinegar rinses have quite dramatic curative properties in some cases. I would suggest that you try the following regime for a month:

➤ Dandruff is often an indication of an overacid body. Try to include lots of fruit and vegetables in your diet. Start the day with the juice of a lemon in a glass of water, and drink lots of water during the day.

➤ Shampoo every third day using the recipe below.

➤ Use a vinegar rinse to follow the shampoo. (Use two bowls—one containing the rinse and the other to catch the drips.) Repeat at least six times.

➤ Use the Anti-dandruff Tonic (recipe at right) every night.

➤ Expose the head to sunlight for at least ten minutes a day (bearing in mind the holes in the ozone layer and skin cancer). The best times of the day to do this safely are before 10 a.m. and after 4 p.m.

➤ Wearing a head covering for extended periods can cause dandruff, so keep the head uncovered as much as possible. This is difficult if you have to wear a safety helmet or similar as part of your job, but just be aware of the problem and remove the hat/helmet as much as possible to let the scalp breathe.

➤ Eat more vitamin B foods (see Chapter Seven). There seems to be a link between vitamin B_6 deficiency and eczema and dandruff.

➤ Be persistent and be positive!

Anti-dandruff Shampoo

Make a shampoo using one of the recipes in this chapter. The herbal decoction should include as many as possible of the following herbs: parsley, lemon grass, mint, nasturtium leaves, lavender, nettle, rosemary and willow bark.

Anti-dandruff Rinse

Make the Herbal Hair Rinse using the same herbs as those in the shampoo. Add 1 teaspoon borax and $^1/_4$ cup (60ml/2fl oz) Herb Vinegar (see Chapter One) to each 2 cups (500ml/16fl oz) of finished rinse. Make sure that the borax is completely dissolved before using.

Anti-dandruff Tonic

The herbs used in the decoction should be the same as those in the Anti-dandruff Shampoo and Rinse (above).

1 teaspoon borax
1 cup (250ml/8fl oz) hot triple strength
infusion/decoction
20 drops rosemary oil
10 drops lavender oil
10 drops tea tree oil
2 teaspoons witch hazel
1 tablespoon cider vinegar

Dissolve the borax and decoction together in a bowl, then allow to cool. Add the remaining ingredients and bottle. Store in the refrigerator. Shake well before use.

Part the hair and rub a little of the tonic onto the scalp using a cotton wool ball. Repeat this all over the scalp. This should be done each night until the problem has been cured.

CHAPTER FOUR

THE BATH

And what a romp they had! The bathroom was
drenched with their splashings.
Of such is the kingdom of heaven.
—**ALDOUS HUXLEY (1894–1963)**

A bathroom can be a special place to 'space out' alone; a

place for fun, privacy and relaxation with a partner; a place

for splashing, laughing, scrubbing, and talking with the

children; or merely a place to get clean. Whichever (or all)

of these you enjoy, you will find recipes in the following

pages which will enhance the experience.

Soap dish from Crabtree & Evelyn

Home-made bath products make a haven in the bath. Herbal infusions
are often used as a base, giving lovely earthy coloured products.

THE BATH

I used to visit a commune where the bath was in the middle of a very beautiful vegetable garden. The water was heated with an ingenious arrangement of large black-painted, 44-gallon drums on stands. Climbing beans formed a living tepee over the path, and melons and pumpkins formed a carpet of bold yellow flowers around the area.

This 'bathroom' led me to fantasise on a garden bathroom of my own, surrounded by fragrant herbs and vines, hanging with grapes within easy reach of my hands. Here I would spend luxurious hours and would surely become enlightened!

The fantasy was destroyed when I visited the commune in the winter. The bath and waterstands were abandoned and work had commenced on what was called (by the local council) an ablutions block. I (and the residents) had overlooked the fact that when there was no sun, the water in the tanks doesn't get hot and it's not very romantic sitting in cold water in a vegetable garden on a cold, wet and windy day surrounded by rotting cabbages!

As I was writing the last paragraph a friend, Fiona Morgan, delivered some copy for the South West Herb Society's magazine, which I edit. I asked her permission to reproduce some of it here and have now begun converting the arbour down the garden into our 'star-gazing' bathroom!

'For many, the humble bath has been replaced with the convenience of the modern-day shower, yet some continue bathing, enjoying the relaxation, 'time-out' behind closed doors.

Bathing took on a new meaning for me when I was working on the Nullarbor Plain. There, we tubbed in the open, in an old enamel bath with a gentle fire burning beneath. The angle for star-gazing is perfect with your neck gently supported by the end of the bath. It was then that I began to discover the universe, and my perception of the world and existence was profoundly changed.

Now, six years on, our bathing ritual has continued with the old enamel tub carefully positioned on the hill where star-gazing is at its best. We ceremoniously light the fire and get the water temperature 'just right'. With embers glowing we can luxuriate (even in the rain) without the water going cold. We have a thick rubber mat to sit on or the bottom of the bath isn't the only thing which would get warm!

Obviously, those with hovering neighbours may feel that this is not for them but we have fellow 'tubbing-mates' in suburbia who've designed special, private, peaceful areas in their gardens, with the bath as the focal point! We often light the fire under our tub for visitors and they usually go home and set their own up as quickly as possible.'

If you can't indulge yourself in an outdoor bathroom then a compromise is to make your bathroom as restful and beautiful as you can—a shelf near at hand for a book, a drink, cassette player (a safe distance away), bath salts and anything else which will make you feel secure and relaxed. Tropical plants add an exotic feel to a bathroom and most of them love living in a bathroom as the air becomes humid and 'jungle-like'.

We take water for granted and overlook the precious gift that it is. Our bodies need it inside and appreciate it outside. Water stimulates, relaxes, heals and purifies. Maurice Messegue, the famous French herbalist, uses hot herbal foot and hand baths in preference to administering herbs internally. He finds that the infusion which is absorbed by the skin into the bloodstream works faster and much more efficiently than the same infusion taken internally and absorbed through the digestive system.

Too frequent bathing or showering can be bad for your skin; it may be great for your nerves or morale but it can strip the skin of needed oils and can produce irritation. We have become increasingly obsessed with body smells, preferring to substitute other smells and/or suppress the natural ones.

There are only a few areas in which the body odour becomes nasty—the feet, armpits, and genital/anal areas. These are the only areas which need soap (unless you have very oily skin, or grimy hands and feet). Don't scrub away at your poor tummy and back as though you are punishing them: unless you are a mud wrestler, these parts will only need warm water to cleanse them. 'Warm' is the key word in the last sentence. Hot water is very destructive to skin. It can result in dryness, irritation, and 'broken' capillary veins and should only be used for therapeutic reasons.

Dry-brush massage is a terrific treatment for your skin. It stimulates the circulation and gets rid of the dead cells which give skin such a 'muddy' look; skin feels very 'alive' after brushing. It's possible to buy inexpensive, long-handled natural bristle brushes at pharmacies and variety stores. Use the brush before your bath or shower and brush in a circular movement all over your body, paying special attention to areas where there are glands, such as the armpits, groin and just below the collarbone. Be gentle on breasts and around the genital area.

Silver shell soap dish, wire soap basket with shells, scent sachet, blue and white checked soap dish, shell box and ceramic soap dish from Linen and Lace of Balmain; shell spoons from The Bay Tree; bath brush and pink floral soap dish from Crabtree & Evelyn; face washers from The Body Shop, flowers by Lisa Milasas

TYPES OF BATHS

HOT BATH

38–40°C (100–104°F); 10–15 minutes only. The effects are increased perspiration and rate of breathing; reduction of fevers; elimination of toxins. Wrap up in blankets after the bath and drink appropriate hot herb teas during and after the bath.

WARM BATH

27–34°C (80–93°F); indulge for 20 minutes to 1 hour. The effects are mild, calming, relaxing.

COLD BATH

21–27°C (69–80°F); 2–5 minutes only. The effects are improved breathing and muscle tone; decreased fatigue; improved thyroid function and skin tone; relief from constipation.

BRAN BATH

Anyone who suffers from dry, itchy skin will enjoy the benefits of a bran bath. You can simply throw a handful of bran in the bath, but as that is really messy, it's better to put a handful in a pan, cover with 3 cups (750ml/24fl oz) of water, bring it to the boil, simmer for a few minutes, then strain the water into the bath. Alternatively, tie a handful of bran in a muslin bag (see Straining and Filtering in Chapter One), squeeze it under the bath water to release the 'milkiness' and then use the bran-filled bag as a washcloth.

BUBBLE BATHS

These are fun and have a luxurious feeling but it's not good to indulge for too long or too often as they are detergent-based and can overdry the skin. Use only the amount recommended and apply moisturiser to your skin after the bath.

EPSOM SALTS

After a long day in the garden my soul is flying but my body feels wrecked. I add half a box of Epsom salts and a few drops of essential oil to a warm bath while the water is running and I soak for at least half an hour. The bath seems to take all the weariness away and leaves me feeling very refreshed.

HERB BATH

There are many suggestions for herb baths throughout this chapter. Herbs may be used to heal, hydrate, soothe, stimulate, relax, soften, tighten and much more. There are many ways to introduce the plants to your bath: infusions; decoctions; bath bags; bath mitts; oils; or combined with any of the other treatments in this section.

HONEY BATH

An old, well-tried and simple skin softener which also helps you to sleep. Mix a tablespoonful of honey with some warm water until it's very runny. Pour into a warm (not hot) bath, swish it around and enjoy!).

MILK BATH

Unless you have access to an ass you will have to be content with adding fresh or powdered milk to your bath water. The protein and other contents of the milk leave the skin feeling silky and soft. Yoghurt or buttermilk give a mildly acidic and protein-enriched bath.

MUSTARD BATH

When you arrive home cold, wet and shivery you can avoid a full-scale cold by having a Mustard Foot bath (see Therapeutic Foot baths in this chapter).

SALT BATH

If you are dirty you might like to have a shower or wash first, as the salt prevents soap lathering. Add 2 teacups of cooking salt to the bath as the water is running. It should be a warm, not hot, bath for the best results. After this bath you will feel fresh, stimulated and silky skinned.

VINEGAR BATH

Another bath to ease itchy skin. You can either slosh in cider vinegar or a Herbal Bath Vinegar (see Bath Vinegars in this chapter).

BATHING
WITH HERBS

Herbs in the bath hydrate and soothe the skin but it's not much fun having a bath with twigs and leaves floating around in it; they will clog your plumbing if not laboriously picked out at the end of your relaxing bath time, destroying the mood and mystique. Much better to use one of the following methods, choose herbs from the Bath Herbs chart.

- Put a handful of herbs in a saucepan, cover with water, add 1–2 tablespoons cider vinegar, cover with a lid and simmer over a low heat for 20 minutes. Strain (put the herbs in your compost bucket) and pour the wonderfully rich herb soup into the bath or sponge it over your body when you have finished showering. The cider vinegar creates the correct acid balance and also extracts more properties from the herbs than water alone.

- Chop the herbs and tie them in a piece of fine cloth or a muslin bag (see Straining and Filtering in Chapter One), hang the bundle under the hot tap as it's running, then use it as a washcloth.

- If you are in a hurry or don't have access to fresh herbs you can use herbal tea bags, either dropped into the bath and squeezed well, or made into a strong infusion which is used the same as the first method, above.

- Bath mitts accompanied by a big jar of herbal mix make a nice gift to use in the bath or shower. To make a mitt you will need towelling—about 20cm x 46cm (8in x 18in). You can use face flannels but that's a bit extravagant as they need trimming. Blanket stitch or machine zigzag along one long edge (this becomes the wrist edge i.e. the mitt's opening). Cut into three mitt shapes, then stitch together around three sides, leaving the previously zigzagged edges free. You now have a mitt with two pockets—one for the herb mixture and one for your hand. If liked you can sew on a loop for hanging the mitt up to dry.

- Less glamorous but as effective are bags made from the feet of pantihose.

Luxury bath products can easily be made in your kitchen and at a fraction of the price of the bought variety. Most of the treatments suggested for the bath may be used in the shower. Do be careful when using essential oils directly into the bath water. I once sprinkled a few drops of rosemary oil on the water but didn't 'swoosh' the water. As I climbed in I must have collected the oil on the calf of my leg and the outside of the thigh. After a few moments I experienced a burning sensation and after the bath I was very red and lightly blistered in these areas. I had been using these oils for decades and should have known better!

The following preparations are for mixtures of dried herbs which are nice in the bath. The quantities are quite large so that you have them ready to give as gifts or keep on hand ready to use. (Fresh herbs are lovely to use as the perfume is usually more intense but, unless you intend to dry the surplus, the recipe should be reduced to an amount suitable for only one bath.)

The essential oils are optional but they intensify both the perfume and the therapeutic effect of the bath. Mix the dried herbs thoroughly, sprinkle the essential oil evenly through the herbs, then mix again.

Powdered dried orris root or clary sage added to these mixtures helps to fix the perfume.

Lemon Refresher bath blend

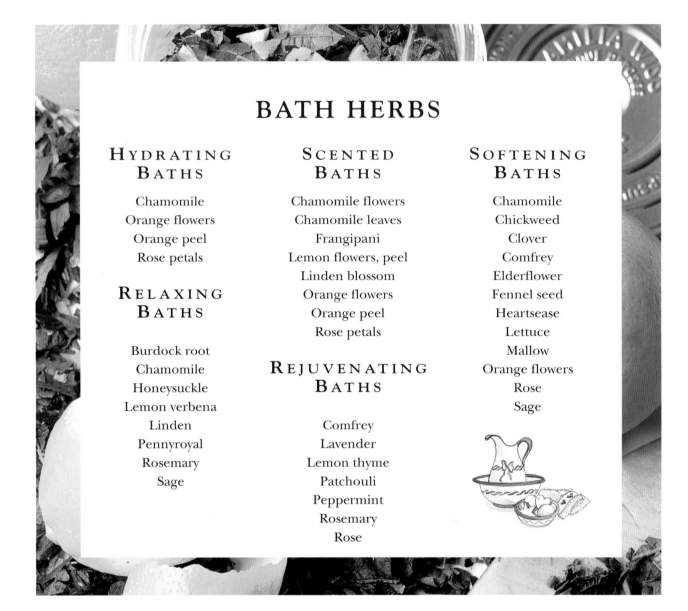

BATH HERBS

HYDRATING BATHS

Chamomile
Orange flowers
Orange peel
Rose petals

RELAXING BATHS

Burdock root
Chamomile
Honeysuckle
Lemon verbena
Linden
Pennyroyal
Rosemary
Sage

SCENTED BATHS

Chamomile flowers
Chamomile leaves
Frangipani
Lemon flowers, peel
Linden blossom
Orange flowers
Orange peel
Rose petals

REJUVENATING BATHS

Comfrey
Lavender
Lemon thyme
Patchouli
Peppermint
Rosemary
Rose

SOFTENING BATHS

Chamomile
Chickweed
Clover
Comfrey
Elderflower
Fennel seed
Heartsease
Lettuce
Mallow
Orange flowers
Rose
Sage

Lemon Refresher

Run the hot water over the dried herb mixture, then add the cold water.

3 teacups dried lemon balm
2 teacups dried lemon verbena
2 tablespoons dried, ground lemon peel
2 tablespoons dried, ground orange peel
$\frac{1}{2}$ teacup dried mint leaves
1 dropper peppermint oil

Crumble the dried herbs until the mixture resembles tea leaves. Drizzle the oil over the mixture while stirring. Store in a tightly sealed container. (If using fresh herbs, prepare a smaller quantity for immediate use.)

Add $\frac{1}{4}$–$\frac{1}{2}$ teacup of the mixture to each bath.

Young Again

If you are feeling old and need a pick-me-up, try this mixture. After your bath you might bounce out of the bathroom, yelling 'Anyone for tennis?'.

3 teacups dried lavender flowers
1 teacup dried rosemary leaves
2 teacups dried peppermint leaves
1 teacup dried comfrey leaves
1 dropper peppermint oil

Crumble the dried herbs until the mixture resembles tea leaves. Drizzle the oil over the mixture while stirring. Store in a tightly sealed container. (If using fresh herbs, prepare a smaller quantity for immediate use.)

Add ¼–½ teacup of the mixture to each bath.

Soft Touch

When your skin feels sore and dry and your mind feels 'scratchy', this bath will make your skin feel like silk, will calm the mind and soothe the heart.

½ teacup bicarbonate of soda
4 teacups rolled oats
2 teacups bran
2 tablespoons wholemeal flour
1 tablespoon borax
1 teacup dried milk
1 dropper lavender oil

Crumble the dried herbs until the mixture resembles tea leaves. Drizzle oil over the mixture while stirring. Store in a tightly sealed container. (If using fresh herbs, prepare a smaller quantity for immediate use.)

Add ¼–½ teacup of the mixture to each bath.

Quickie Herbal Bath

Use herbal tea bags to make a very strong brew. Tip it in the bath and fold the used bags in a piece of cheesecloth to use as a body washer.

Silk Touch

Here is another mixture which hydrates the skin, leaving it soft and pliable.

2 teacups dried crushed chamomile flowers
½ teacup dried crushed orange flowers
1 teacup dried ground orange peel
2 teacups dried crushed rose petals
1 teacup dried, powdered mallow or comfrey root
1 dropper chamomile or orange oil

Crumble the dried herbs until the mixture resembles tea leaves. Drizzle the oil over the mixture while stirring. Store in a tightly sealed container. (If using fresh herbs, prepare a smaller quantity for immediate use.)

Add ¼–½ teacup of the mixture to each bath.

Deodorant

Gently deodorising for a sweet-smelling body.

2 teacups dried lovage root, finely chopped
2 teacups dried crushed lavender flowers
½ teacup dried crushed rosemary leaves
1 teacup dried crushed sage leaves
½ teacup dried crushed thyme leaves
¼ dropper patchouli oil
¼ dropper orange oil

Crumble the dried herbs until the mixture resembles tea leaves. Drizzle the oils over the mixture while stirring. Store in a tightly sealed container. (If using fresh herbs, prepare a smaller quantity for immediate use.)

Add ¼–½ teacup of the mixture to each bath.

Relaxing and Soothing

Try this bath to soothe the nerves after a hectic day.

2 teacups dried chamomile flowers
2 teacups dried honeysuckle flowers
½ teacup dried sage leaves
1 teacup dried rosemary leaves
1 dropper lavender oil

Crumble the dried herbs until the mixture resembles tea leaves. Drizzle the oil over the mixture while stirring. Store in a tightly sealed container. (If using fresh herbs, prepare a smaller quantity for immediate use.)

Add ¼–½ teacup of the mixture to each bath.

The Softie

This bath mixture will soften and hydrate rough or dry skin.

½ teacup dried chamomile flowers
1 teacup dried comfrey leaves
½ teacup dried comfrey root, ground
¼ cup dried mallow root, ground
2 cups dried soapwort root, leaves
and stems, ground
1 teacup dried elderflowers
½ teacup borax

Crumble the dried herbs until the mixture resembles tea leaves. Stir in the borax well. Store in a tightly sealed container. (If using fresh herbs, prepare a smaller quantity for immediate use.)

Add ¼–½ teacup of the mixture to each bath.

Zinger

Rosemary and hyssop have a reputation as brain medicines so if you suffer from brain fag try this bath mixture.

1 teacup dried hyssop leaves
1 teacup dried rosemary leaves
1 teacup dried southernwood leaves
1 teacup dried lemon balm

Crumble the dried herbs until the mixture resembles tea leaves. Stir well. Store in a tightly sealed container. (If using fresh herbs, prepare a smaller quantity for immediate use.)

Add ¼–½ teacup of the mixture to each bath.

Rosie Mist

For romantic evenings, this sensual, sensuous bath blend evokes memories of moonlight and violins!

2 teacups dried scented rose petals
2 teacups dried rose geranium leaves
½ teacup dried lavender (leaves and flowers)
½ teacup dried patchouli
1 dropper ylang-ylang or jasmine oil

Crumble the dried herbs until the mixture resembles tea leaves. Drizzle the oil over the mixture while stirring. Store in a tightly sealed container. (If using fresh herbs, prepare a smaller quantity for immediate use.)

Add ¼–½ teacup of the mixture to each bath.

Bowl and jars from The Bay Tree; jug from Linen and Lace of Balmain; flowers by Lisa Milasas

Rosie Mist bath blend made using fresh rose petals

Sleepy-time Bath

This will help to ensure a good night's sleep. The bath should be warm, not hot. Sip a cup of chamomile/catnep tea sweetened with honey while relaxing in the bath. After you have soaked for 20–30 minutes, dry your body gently and slip between the sheets.

3 teacups dried catnep
2 teacups dried chamomile flowers
½ teacup dried hop flowers
1 tablespoon borax

Crumble the dried herbs until the mixture resembles tea leaves. Stir in the borax well. Store in a tightly sealed container. (If using fresh herbs, prepare a smaller quantity for immediate use.)

Add ¼–½ teacup of the mixture to each bath.

'Flora'

Flora and the country green.
Dance, and Provencal song, and sun-burnt mirth!
— **JOHN KEATS (1795–1821)**

A sweet-smelling mixture which can be used in muslin bath bags or made into a cologne. Packaged in a beautiful bottle, this bath cologne makes a lovely gift.

½ teacup dried peppermint leaves
½ teacup crushed bay leaves
1 teacup dried lemon balm
1 teacup dried lavender
¼ teacup dried wormwood leaves
½ teacup dried marjoram
¼ teacup dried thyme
¼ teacup dried lemon thyme
½ teacup dried angelica, leaf and stem
1 teacup dried scented rose petals
½ dropper lavender oil
½ dropper peppermint oil
2 cups (500ml/16fl oz) vodka or alcohol

Gently simmer the herbs in 2 litres (3½ pints) water in a covered saucepan for 10 minutes. Strain. Repeat the process, using fresh herbs in the strained infusion. Add extra water to bring the amount of infusion back up to 2 litres (3½ pints). Allow to stand for 24 hours. Strain through several layers of cheesecloth. Add the essential oils and alcohol to the infusion. Bottle.

Pour ¼ cup (60ml/2fl oz) into the bath while it's running.

BATH VINEGARS

Nothing is cheaper, easier or more satisfying to make than herbal vinegars. Vinegar restores the acid mantle to skin, relieves dryness, itching and the pain of sunburn. Cider vinegar seems to have the most therapeutic properties but a good quality white vinegar is all right to use. For skin tonics, white wine vinegar is more gentle and refined. If you really hate the smell of vinegar you can substitute vodka (mixed equally with water) or white wine. These last two are more expensive but the perfume of the herb mixture is much more apparent.

The bath herbal vinegars listed below may also be used as:

➤ Hair rinses (add ½ cup (125ml/4fl oz) bath vinegar to 1 litre (32fl oz) water)
➤ Skin tonics (add 1 tablespoon bath vinegar to ½ cup (125ml/4fl oz) water)
➤ After-shower skin friction rub (add ½ cup (125ml/4fl oz) herbal bath vinegar to 1 cup (250ml/8fl oz) water, and avoid all the tender bits!)
➤ Deodorant (use undiluted)

HERBAL BATH VINEGAR

LAVENDER   Traditional, simple and delicate
CITRUS SENSATION   Lemon verbena, lemon thyme, powdered lemon peel, powdered orange peel
MINT TANG   Peppermint, spearmint, apple mint, bruised cloves
HERB SPICE   Sage, rosemary, fennel seeds, star anise
FOREST FANTASY   Pine needles, white oak bark, hyssop, cedar, lemon gum, peppermint
DEODORANT   Lovage, witch hazel bark, sage, white willow bark
SOOTHER FOR ITCHY SKIN   Calendula, chamomile, mallow and comfrey root
FLESH FIRMER!   Horsetail, nettle and honey
SLEEPY TIME   Valerian root, hop flowers, lime flowers, passionfruit flowers, chamomile

Fill a screw-topped jar loosely with the chopped leaves or flowers of your choice, using the list above as a guide.

Pour over vinegar or vodka to cover. Leave for 2 weeks, shaking twice daily (this is important to release the properties from the plant to the liquid.) At the end of the 2 weeks, strain through a sieve or, if not strong enough, repeat the process, then strain through several layers of cheesecloth, and bottle.

Add a dropperful of an appropriate essential oil, if desired. If giving as a gift you can put a sprig of the plant in the bottle as decoration.

Add ¼–½ cup (60–125ml/2–4fl oz) bath vinegar to the bath water.

BUBBLES, OILS AND CREAMS

BUBBLE BATHS

There are few bath treatments which are as much fun or feel as luxurious as a bubble bath. How often do we see films with glamorous actors, champagne glass in hand, lounging indolently in circular marble baths with bubbles coyly hiding all but the head and shoulders?

Bubble baths are detergent-based and can overdry the skin, so one should not indulge for too long or too often. Use only the amount recommended. The base of most commercial bubble baths is the cheapest available detergent. You can make your own superior product by using a good shampoo or the very best quality detergent available.

It's good to use a massage oil or moisture lotion after the bath to counteract the drying effects. The addition of honey, glycerine or oil to recipes also counteracts the drying effect of the detergent.

Protein Bubble Bath

2 teaspoons powdered gelatine
2 tablespoons very hot water
1 cup (250ml/8fl oz) good quality shampoo or detergent
4 droppers essential oils of choice
1 tablespoon glycerine

Sprinkle the gelatine over the water and stir until dissolved. Add the remaining ingredients and mix well. Bottle.

Slowly trickle $^{1}/_{4}$–$^{1}/_{2}$ cup (60–125ml/2–4fl oz) of the mixture under a fast-running tap to maximise the bubbles.

'Orange Grove' Bubble Bath

$^{1}/_{4}$ cup (60ml/2fl oz) canola oil
1 cup (250ml/8fl oz) good quality shampoo or detergent
1 dropper petitgrain oil
1 dropper lemon oil
1 dropper orange oil
1 dropper sandalwood oil

Combine all the ingredients, then bottle. Slowly trickle $^{1}/_{4}$ cup (60ml/2fl oz) of the mixture under a fast-running tap to maximise the bubbles.

Golden Bubbles

$^{1}/_{2}$ cup (125ml/4fl oz) good quality golden-coloured shampoo or detergent
1 egg, beaten
1 teaspoon honey
1 teaspoon glycerine
1 dropper essential oil of choice

Combine all the ingredients together then bottle. Slowly trickle $^{1}/_{4}$ cup (60ml/2fl oz) of the mixture under a fast-running tap to maximise the bubbles.

Enamel dish from The Bay Tree; timber bath mat from Linen and Lace of Balmain; flowers by Lisa Milasas

Making Golden Bubbles

BATH OILS

Bath oils are dispersible, semi-dispersible and floating. As the names suggest, the dispersible oils dissolve entirely into the bath water, semi-dispersible mostly dissolve into the water and non-dispersible float on the top.

There are advantages to all three types. Sometimes if my skin feels dry I like the sensation of the oil clinging to my body as I step into the bath and of the 'blobs' of oil which float towards me and settle on my skin as I sit in the bath. The disadvantage of this type of bath oil is that the 'blobs' cling to the sides of the bath as well as to your skin, and you need to spend time after the bath both massaging it into your skin and cleaning it off the bath!

Use the Herb Oil Base (see Chapter One) in these recipes to get maximum benefits.

Dispersible oils frequently contain alcohol but in such small quantities that there is no danger of drying the skin.

HERB OIL BASE: HOT METHOD

For more information on Herb Oil Bases see Chapter One.

This method will make a triple strength oil.

1   Place the minced herbs in a crock-pot or double boiler and cover with oil.

2   Add 1 tablespoon cider vinegar to each litre (32fl oz) of oil, and stir well. Cover with a lid and leave for 1–2 hours. The vinegar extracts properties left behind by the oil and also helps to speed up the extraction.

3   Keeping the cover on, heat gently to no more than 45–48°C (113–118°F); if the oil overheats you will lose some of the important volatile properties of the herbs. When the temperature is reached, turn the heat off and allow to cool.

4   Repeat stage 3 several times over a period of 24 hours.

5   Strain the oil through cheesecloth, squeezing the bag to extract as much oil as possible. If you want a single strength oil you can go to stage 7.

6   To make triple strength oil you need to repeat stages 1–5 twice more, using the original oil each time but topping up with fresh oil to keep the quantity the same.

7   Pour the finished oil into a jar. After a few days you will see sediment at the bottom of the jar. Carefully decant the oil into a clean jar, leaving the sediment behind. Refrigerate the oil until needed. I refrigerate the sediment and use it in packs and masks.

'Waters of Babylon' Bath Oil

This bath oil is dispersible. Use within 2 weeks.

2 eggs
1 tablespoon cider vinegar
¼ cup (60ml/2fl oz) vodka
1 tablespoon glycerine
1 cup (250ml/8fl oz) Herb Oil Base
1 teaspoon essential oil
1 tablespoon good quality detergent

Beat the first 4 ingredients together in a bowl. Drizzle in the herb and essential oil, still beating. Stir in the detergent thoroughly, then bottle. Keep refrigerated.

Add ¼ cup (60ml/2fl oz) to the bath as the water is running.

Citrus Moisturising Bath Oil

This bath oil is dispersible and keeps well without refrigeration.

½ cup (125ml/4fl oz) vodka
2 teaspoons lemon oil
1 teaspoon orange oil
¼ teaspoon clove oil
1 tablespoon tincture of benzoin
60g (2oz) lanolin
1 tablespoon runny honey
1½ cups (375ml/12fl oz) Herb Oil Base

Dissolve the vodka, oils and tincture together in a bowl. Heat the lanolin, honey and herb oil in a small saucepan. Don't overheat. Take off the heat, slowly add to the vodka mixture while stirring constantly. Bottle.

Add ¼ cup (60ml/2fl oz) to the bath as the water is running.

Sunset Bath Oil

This is a silky and moisturising bath oil. It is semi-dispersible and keeps for about 3 weeks if refrigerated. See Chapter One for hints on mixing pectin. Other gelling agents may be used if liked.

2 rounded teaspoons pectin powder
⅓ cup (80ml/2⅔fl oz) vodka
2 cups (500ml/16fl oz) triple strength herbal infusion
2 tablespoons glycerine
¼ cup (60ml/2fl oz) Herb Oil Base
1 teaspoon geranium oil
1 teaspoon ylang-ylang oil

Mix the pectin and vodka together until smooth. Add the remaining ingredients very slowly to the above, stirring constantly to mix. Bottle.

Add 1–2 tablespoons to the bath as the water is running.

Herbal Bath Oil

This semi-dispersible bath oil keeps indefinitely if refrigerated.

1 cup (250ml/8fl oz) Herb Oil Base
¼ cup (60ml/2fl oz) herbal shampoo
1 teaspoon rosemary oil
1 teaspoon geranium oil
½ teaspoon bergamot oil
½ teaspoon patchouli oil

Mix all the ingredients together in a bottle. About 2 tablespoons added to the bath while the water is running should be enough unless you want to make the bath water very bubbly.

Aromatherapy Bath Oil

Choose the oils for this semi-dispersible bath oil from the table on Essential Oils for Skin in Chapter Two. You may need a therapeutic action or a perfume to appeal to the senses, or feel that you need spiritually uplifting. Whatever you want will be available to you through the magic of essential oils.

1 cup (250ml/8fl oz) brandy or vodka
5 teaspoons essential oils
3 teaspoons glycerine

Place all the ingredients in a bottle and shake very well.

One teaspoonful will be plenty for this bath—any more and you might overdose on the powerful fragrance or you might become enlightened and float off the planet!

Floating Bath Oil

1 cup (250ml/8fl oz) Herb Oil Base
3 teaspoons essential oil of choice

Place all the ingredients in a bottle and shake well.

Try 1 tablespoon added to the bath at first, as it's easy to add too much and then to feel as though you are in the centre of an oceanic oil spill. After the bath, massage any clinging oil into the skin.

Ingredients used in making bath oils

Spice Satin

This lovely, dispersible, bath oil will keep for a long time if stored in the refrigerator. Men particularly like it as it smells more masculine than some of the other recipes. Any of the mucilages in Chapter One may be used but the quantities will need to be adapted as each has different thickening properties.

2 tablespoons vodka
2 tablespoons pectin powder
2 cups (500ml/16fl oz) warm water
1½ tablespoons olive oil
1½ tablespoons almond oil
20 drops cinnamon oil
10 drops clove oil
1 teaspoon vanilla essence

Mix the vodka and pectin powder together in a bowl. Add the water slowly, beating well until there are no lumps. Leave to thicken for a few hours.

Beat the remaining ingredients together, then slowly mix into the pectin mixture. Add more water if the mixture is too thick. Store in the refrigerator.

Add about ¼–½ cup (60–125ml/2–4fl oz) to the bath as it's running.

Lavender Soother

This satin mixture will ease a body sore from the sun. The oil disperses in the water.

2 tablespoons pectin powder
2 tablespoons vodka
2 cups (500ml/16fl oz) warm water
1 tablespoon glycerine
¼ cup (60ml/2fl oz) castor oil
30 drops lavender oil
10 drops clove oil

Mix the pectin and vodka together in a bowl. Slowly beat the water and glycerine into the pectin mixture. Leave for a few hours to thicken. Slowly beat in the remaining ingredients until blended. Store in the refrigerator.

Add ½ cup (125ml/4fl oz) of this satin mixture to a warm bath and splash over the 'scorched' bits.

White glass dish from The Bay Tree; tea towels from Linen and Lace of Balmain; flowers by Lisa Milasas

Making Lavender Soother bath oil, a soothing blend for sunburn

BATH CREAMS

These creams need refrigeration and should be used within 2 weeks. They are easy to make and leave the skin soft and moisturised. Don't add them to very hot water or the egg will set and go stringy. The oil disperses in the water and doesn't leave a greasy ring around the bath.

Grapefruit and Honey Cream

1 egg
½ cup (125ml/4fl oz) canola oil
2 teaspoons glycerine
2 teaspoons runny honey
½ teacup dried milk powder
20 drops grapefruit oil
10 drops lemon oil
10 drops orange oil
2 cups (500ml/16fl oz) water

Beat the egg, canola oil, glycerine, honey and milk powder together in a bowl. Add the essential oils while still beating. Beat the water in, a little at a time. Store in the refrigerator.

Add ¼–½ cup (60–125ml/2–4fl oz) to the bath water.

Cinnamon Cream

1 egg
¼ cup (60ml/2fl oz) canola oil
¼ cup (60ml/2fl oz) olive oil
1 tablespoon runny honey
20 drops cinnamon oil
10 drops clove oil
10 drops vanilla essence
2 teaspoons gelatine powder
2 cups (500ml/16fl oz) very hot water

Beat the canola oil, olive oil, honey and cinnamon oil together in a bowl. Add the clove oil and vanilla while beating. Sprinkle the gelatine over the hot water and stir until dissolved. Beat the gelatine mixture slowly into the oil mixture until well combined. Store in the refrigerator.

Add ¼–½ cup (60–125ml/2–4fl oz) to the bath water.

BATH SALTS

Bath salts are used primarily to soften hard water and may also contain essential oils to perfume the water and add therapeutic properties. If you would like to colour the salts you can add a few drops of natural colouring drop by drop after adding the oils.

Temple Chimes

200g (6½oz) tartaric acid
200g (6½oz) bicarbonate of soda
100g (3⅓oz) arrowroot powder
10 drops frankincense oil
20 drops cypress oil
5 drops sandalwood oil
5 drops patchouli oil

Mix the dry ingredients together. Add the mixed oils drop by drop, stirring all the time to prevent caking. Place the mixture in a jar and shake daily for a few days.

Sprinkle ¼–½ teacup of the mixture into the bath as it is running.

Bay Salt Bath

This scrub will thoroughly cleanse the skin.

bay leaves, bruised
cooking salt

Layer the bay leaves and salt together in a large jar and leave for 1 month.

Wet your body in the shower. Turn off the water and scrub your body gently with a handful of the salt. Avoid the genital area. After the scrub, step into a bathful of warm water which has been perfumed and softened with one of the bath oil recipes. If your shower is over the bath, rinse off the salt under the shower and massage in a massage oil found in Chapter Six.

Refreshing, Rejuvenating Mineral Bath

200g (6½oz) Epsom salts
100g (3⅓oz) sea salt
2 tablespoons bicarbonate of soda
1 tablespoon tartaric acid
2 tablespoons cornflour
40 drops lavender oil
20 drops clove oil

Mix all the dry ingredients together. Add the essential oils drop by drop, stirring all the time. Place the mixture in a jar and stir twice daily for a few days.

Sprinkle ¼ teacup of the mixture in the bath as it is running.

Desert Island Dream

This is luscious. Use the type of coconut oil used for flavouring chocolate (not the same as coconut fixed oil which has no scent).

100g (3⅓oz) tartaric acid
100g (3⅓oz) bicarbonate of soda
60g (2oz) arrowroot powder
coconut oil as required (not more than 40 drops)

Mix all the dry ingredients together well. Add the coconut oil until the scent is as strong as you desire. Place the mixture in a jar and shake daily for a few days.

Sprinkle ¼ teacup of the mixture into the bath as it is running.

Green Wave Bath Salts

This blend smells of the Australian bush and the ocean—very bracing and refreshing.

200g (6½oz) bicarbonate of soda
60g (2oz) tartaric acid
1 teacup Irish moss, ground to a powder
3 teacups sea salt
40 drops pine oil
40 drops cypress oil
20 drops eucalyptus oil

Mix all the dry ingredients together. Add the essential oils drop by drop, stirring all the time. Place the mixture in a jar and shake daily for a few days.

Sprinkle ½ teacup of the mixture into the bath as it is running.

THERAPEUTIC FOOT BATHS

Baths can be used for many purposes other than cleanliness and pleasure. Skin is capable of absorbing herbal decoctions, infusions and essential oils and can therefore become a valuable part of any therapeutic treatment.

The following baths are just a few suggestions for mixtures which may be used to alleviate medical conditions. Essential oils may also be used as a substitute for herbs or combined with herbs to enhance the action.

For further information on foot baths, see Foot Care in Chapter Two.

For Coughs

thyme leaves
aniseeds
peppermint leaves
tea tree leaves

Choose a bowl with enough room for both feet. Make sufficient triple strength infusion/decoction from the herbs to half fill the foot bath bowl. (For instructions on making an infusion/decoction, see Chapter One.) Have the liquid as hot as can be borne and immerse the feet for a minimum of 15 minutes. Top up with boiling water (carefully!) if the mixture cools off too much.

For Headache

basil
lavender
linden
marjoram

Choose a bowl with enough room for both feet. Make sufficient triple strength infusion/decoction from the herbs to half fill the foot bath bowl. (For instructions on making an infusion/decoction, see Chapter One.) Have the liquid as hot as can be borne and immerse the feet for a minimum of 15 minutes. Top up with boiling water (carefully!) if the mixture cools off too much.

For Influenza

1 teaspoon chilli powder
elderflower flowers
peppermint leaves
yarrow flowers and leaves

Mix the chilli powder to a paste with a little water and thoroughly stir into the hot foot bath water. Make a very hot infusion of the herbs and sip it while soaking the feet for 15 minutes. Go directly to bed after the treatment.

Head Cold or Pre-cold 'Shivery Feeling'

2 teaspoons mustard powder
elderflower flowers
peppermint leaves
yarrow flowers and leaves

Mix the mustard powder to a paste with a little water and stir it into the hot foot bath water. Make a very hot infusion of the herbs and sip it while soaking the feet for 15 minutes. Go directly to bed after the treatment.

Face washers from The Body Shop; tin basin and soap dish from Linen and Lace of Balmain; bath brush and mit from Crabtree & Evelyn; flowers by Lisa Milasas

An exotic therapeutic foot bath

AFTER-BATH POWDERS

Excessive use of powder is not recommended as it has the effect of blocking the pores. However there are occasions when it feels cool and comfortable to apply a light dusting of delicately perfumed gossamer powder to your body or feet.

In addition to the recipes below, you will find baby powders and other deodorant powders in Chapter Two.

As a base powder, you can choose from arrowroot, cornflour or talcum powder. If using the latter, use only pharmaceutical-standard, sterilised talcum powder (see Glossary).

Floral Mist Bath Powder

One of my favourite herbs to use in this mixture is oakmoss. I love its tender, gentle and musky perfume which blends well with orris and violet.

250g (8oz) base powder (see above)
30g (1oz) orris root (see Glossary)
dried, crushed, perfumed flowers and herbs
dried citrus peel
crushed cinnamon stick

Combine all the ingredients in a jar, stir daily and leave to mature for as long as it takes. When the mixture smells breathtakingly beautiful, it's ready. Sieve through a coarse and then a fine sieve and pack in shallow boxes or dishes with lids or in recycled sprinkle/puffer packs.

Deodorant Powder

250g (8oz) talcum
30g (1oz) orris root (see Glossary)
dried and crushed lovage, patchouli, rosemary, thyme, lavender
dried, powdered orange peel
finely crushed myrrh

Combine all the ingredients in a wide-mouthed jar. Stir daily until the perfume is pronounced. Sieve through a coarse and then a fine sieve. Package in boxes or jars.

Aromatherapy Powder

The basic powder may be perfumed by the addition of essential oils. Add the oils a drop at a time until the perfume is as strong as you like. Stir constantly during this process or lumps will develop in the powder. The addition of orris powder will stabilise the perfume. Keep the powder in a wide-mouthed jar for a week or so and stir or shake daily to distribute the perfume oils and prevent 'caking'. For oil blends, see Chapter Six.

The following pages, 136 and 137, show ingredients often used in making bath products

A NOTE ON BATH CRYSTALS

Many books suggest that you can make bath crystals at home by colouring and scenting washing soda crystals (the main ingredient in commercial bath crystals). After lengthy discussions with chemists who manufacture washing soda, I really can't recommend the use of this product as bath crystals. A 1% solution has a pH of 11 which would burn really badly; a quarter of a cupful in a bath would be harmless but children usually prefer quantity to quality and would be likely to pour the entire contents of the jar into the bath with possibly disastrous results to the child's skin (irritation and/or burns).

I was told that sodium sesquicarbonate, a much milder water softener, is made by mixing washing soda (sodium carbonate) with sodium bicarbonate. (It was also explained to me that making a saturated solution of either sodium carbonate or sesquicarbonate would result in very beautiful needle-like crystals!) For a description of washing soda, see Glossary.

CHAPTER FIVE

SOAPS

Myths tell of a hill called Sapo near Rome where the Romans sacrificed animals to their gods. The fat from slaughtered animals combined with ash from the fire and ran down the hill to the river below, where the washerwomen worked. The women found that the ash and fat combination made their work much easier.

Soap dish from Crabtree & Evelyn

Home-made soaps can be made in any shape or size

MAKING SOAP

It seems that soap has been around since about 1000 BC. It is created by a process called 'saponification', which happens when a fatty acid (such as tallow or oil) and an alkali (caustic soda) are melted and blended together.

The first time I made soap I was frankly very nervous. My friend Nirala came to help me and we spent the best part of a morning drinking tea and eyeing the container of caustic soda with mounting suspicion. We had both read so many cautions regarding caustic soda (lye) that we had a less than enthusiastic approach. We finally took courage and began, writing in a book everything we did (Nirala is a Virgo and very meticulous).

Since these first experiments I have made lots of soap and there is little to compare with the excitement of turning unpromising and primitive lumps of fat and raw caustic soda into sophisticated and elegant bars of soap.

Glycerine is a by-product of soap making. In the commercial manufacture of soap the glycerine is removed and sold as a separate product. Home-made soap, if well made, is superior to a bought soap as it retains the emollient glycerine.

When you have gained confidence from making a test batch you will be ready to double or quadruple the quantities and try some additives. It's possible to make a fairly large batch and divide it into four, adding different oils, fillers, colours or perfumes to each quarter. It's good to do this with a friend, as you have to work fast.

Following are the basic ingredients, with warnings, quantities and methods. You will find many recipes in this chapter.

CAUTIONS

- Never pour water over caustic soda. When caustic soda is added to cold water the temperature rises almost immediately to about 90–95°C (194–204°F). The caustic must always be added to the water. If the water is poured over the caustic, you might either create a 'hot spot' which could crack or melt the container or there could even be an explosion!
- Never put caustic soda into aluminium—it eats it!
- Never leave your flesh exposed. Wear rubber gloves, long sleeves and shoes.
- Never have children or pets around when you are using caustic soda. Choose a time when the children are elsewhere. Put pets in a separate room.
- Never breathe-in the fumes. Every effort should be made to avoid inhalation. Work in a well ventilated room.
- If the caustic is swallowed, use vinegar or milk as an antidote. DON'T INDUCE VOMITING. Get professional help quickly.
- You will need to have a bottle of vinegar and some cotton wool at hand to neutralise the alkaline, if you get a splash of the caustic liquid or a grain of dry caustic on your skin. After neutralising, wash the area thoroughly with cold water.

WATER

The quality of water used in soap making is very important as hard water contains minerals which can interfere with the action of the lye and your soap will be a failure. The best water to use is either clean rainwater or purified water.

CAUSTIC SODA (LYE)

The Martindale Pharmacopoeia describes caustic soda (sodium hydroxide) as a 'strongly alkaline and corrosive substance which can rapidly destroy tissue'. I made an awestruck comment about this to my friend Fred, the pharmacist, who said, 'Oh, it's not that bad—you've got 5 to 10 seconds to get to a running tap'. This comment didn't increase my confidence at all!

Don't be put off making soap by the cautionary notes. Once you are familiar with this substance and learn to treat it with respect there should be no problems.

FATS AND OILS

Most commercial soaps use animal fats in soap making. It is, however, possible to produce a very good soap using coconut and other oils. The initial quality of the fat used will determine the finished quality of the soap. If you use discoloured smelly fat you will get discoloured smelly soap!

Here is a list of some fats and oils and the types of soap produced from them:

BEEF FAT   Produces hard, white long-lasting soap with small dense bubbles. Needs the addition of some oils to make a fine, easier, lathering soap. Beef fat is known as 'tallow' after rendering.

MUTTON AND LAMB FAT   Produces hard, brittle soap with small bubbles. Best used in conjunction with other fats.

CHICKEN FAT   Too soft on its own but may be used in small quantities with other fats.

PORK FAT   Too soft to use alone. Mix with other fats.

COCONUT OIL   May be used alone but makes a very skin-drying soap. The soap has nice big fat bubbles and will create a lather even in sea water. To gain the best advantage from coconut oil it should be mixed with other fats or oils.

COPHA   This is the trade name of a hydrogenated coconut oil. It is much cheaper than coconut oil and I have found it to be good for soap making.

SUPAFRY   A hydrogenated blend of animal and vegetable fats. It's very easy to use and makes a good soap.

There are many other solid (hydrogenated) frying fats available. I recommend that you use them to make only small quantities of soap until you know how each one behaves.

Oils which add creaminess and skin-softening properties to soaps include: almond oil, canola oil, castor oil, olive oil, palm oil, peanut oil, sesame oil, and wheat germ oil.

TO TREAT FAT FOR SOAP MAKING

Ask your butcher to sell you some clean beef fat, preferably the hard white fat from around the kidneys—1kg (2lb) of fat will reduce to about 500g (1lb) of tallow, so work out in advance how much soap you want to make.

The process may be done on the stove top using a large, deep pan but there is a danger of burning the fat and also the smell is diabolical!

Some books suggest putting the chopped-up fat in water and extracting the tallow by simmering. The water/fat is then strained and cooled until the fat floats on the water in a hard mass. I have tried this method and found it disagreeable, smelly and messy, and the finished fat doesn't feel as hard as the oven method.

Tallow Preparation —Oven Method

Preheat the oven to 160°C (320°F).

Trim the bits of blood, meat or discoloration from the fat and chop it into pieces about the size of small walnuts or less.

Put the fat in a deep baking dish and then in the oven. Leave for several hours or until there is a lot of clear fat with bits of crispy skin and gristle floating in it.

Strain through several layers of cheesecloth into a heatproof container, and when cool and set, store in the refrigerator where it will keep well for a few weeks.

EQUIPMENT NEEDED TO MAKE SOAP

Preserving or laboratory thermometer (not essential but makes the process much easier and more reliable)

Rubber gloves

Apron

Stainless steel tablespoon or really clean wooden spoon

Small heatproof glass measuring jug (e.g. Pyrex) for lye (caustic soda)

Large bowl (glass, plastic, stainless steel or unchipped enamel)

Measuring spoons

Measuring cups

Dieter's scales

Rubber spatula

Moulds

Jar of water for soaking spoons, spatulas etc.

Portable icebox or polystyrene box (e.g. an 'Esky' or something similar)

MATERIALS NEEDED TO MAKE SOAP

Rainwater, purified or distilled water

Caustic soda

Clean tallow

Oil, such as olive oil

Petroleum jelly

Essential oils and other additives (optional)

MEASURING

Standard metric measuring cups and spoons should be used as there is too much variation in ordinary household cutlery and crockery.

I use scales for measuring but here are some conversions for those of you who prefer metric cups and spoons:

caustic soda	$\frac{1}{2}$ cup = 125g (4oz)
caustic soda	1 teaspoon = 5g
water	1 cup = 250ml (8fl oz)
water	1 teaspoon = 5ml
melted fat or oil	1 cup = 250ml (8fl oz)
melted fat or oil	1 teaspoon = 5ml

Green glass from The Bay Tree

Ingredients and equipment needed for soap-making— note the prepared tallow in the large white bowl

ADDITIVES

You will see from the recipes in this book that many additives may be made to soap. These additions should never constitute more than 20% of the total fats. These extras (see below) are usually added just before the soap is ready to pour. If they are added too soon the caustic either destroys or radically changes them.

➤ To add emollient properties: Honey; lecithin; additional oils; lanolin (wool fat); dried milk; egg yolks, glycerine; cold cream.

➤ To create a mildly abrasive but softening soap: Ground oats or bran; ground almonds; cornmeal.

➤ To make soaps to clean dirty and greasy hands: Pumice; sugar; sand.

COLOURING SOAP

Colouring and perfuming soap using natural materials is quite difficult as many colours and scents change or fade radically in the presence of caustic soda.

Commercial soap manufacturers rely on synthetic colours and perfumes which have often been devised specifically for soap making. Many of these synthetics are potential irritants or can produce allergic-type reactions (another good reason for making your own soap).

Many colours extracted from plants lose their vivid blues, reds, greens and yellows and become a disappointing beige when incorporated in the soap mixture. The most predictable and safest colours to use are those found in various spices. The ground spice should be mixed with enough oil to make a thin cream before adding to the 'almost ready to pour' soap. Mix really well to incorporate. Don't add more than 2–3 teaspoons ground spice to each 400g (13oz) of tallow/oil mix or the smell/colour may be too intense. Some of the best colours are obtained from the following spices.

➤ Paprika or annatto: Lovely shades of salmony pinks to reds. Annatto is available from Asian food stores.

➤ Turmeric, saffron or curry powder: Shades of gold to peach.

➤ Cloves, cinnamon or caramel colouring: A wide range from beige to chocolate colour.

➤ Laundry blue: If you shake the powder into the still liquid soap until the soap turns navy blue (about 1–2 tablespoons to 400g (13oz) of soap) you will end up with a pretty lilac colour.

PERFUMING SOAP

Perfuming soap can be as tricky as adding colour. You may be disappointed with the depth of perfume of the finished soap as, even if you added the oil right at the end, the alkali might kill all but the 'bottom notes'.

'Double batching' is a way of getting round the problem—this means that you virtually make the soap twice. It is time-consuming but gives a truer perfume. In the first making and partial curing, the alkali is used up and the saponification completed. Never use synthetic perfume and only 2–3% of the total volume essential oil should be added as these oils are very powerful in their action.

To 'double batch' for the first time you should try the small test quantity (recipe follows) until you are confident.

Perfumed Soap: Test Batch

Grate the soap finely with a plastic or stainless steel grater.

Melt the grated soap with quarter its volume of water in a steel or china bowl over boiling water until it's all dissolved.

Simmer until the soap hangs from the spoon in 'ropes'. (This may take a long time—up to a couple of hours.)

Take from the heat and stand until cooled to about 40°C (104°F).

Add 2–3% (of the total volume) essential oil and mix really well to incorporate the oil before pouring into moulds.

Allow to cure for 1 week.

MOULDS

Almost anything suitably shaped may be used as a soap mould. Aluminium containers should never be used.

Some suggestions: waxed milk cartons; wooden and plastic boxes; soap dishes and the base of plastic soap boxes; individual plastic jelly moulds; cut-down shoe boxes (children's size are the best); individual pâté dishes (straight-sided); individual yoghurt containers. You will find many more ideas as you look around your kitchen or bathroom.

Shoe boxes are my least favourite moulds as the sides tend to bulge, giving the finished soap a poor shape.

If you are using an enclosed container such as a milk carton you will need to tear the carton away carefully from the soap after 4–5 hours as blocks of soap need to be cut before they become too hard. Similarly, if a shoe box or plastic box is used, the soap should be cut into squares when it's still the consistency of hard butter.

Remember that liquid and fresh soap is caustic and will damage varnish, paint, or other colour—this colour might transfer itself to your soap and ruin it. A shoe box or other unwaxed cardboard box should be lined with damp cloth to help prevent the soap leaking through.

WRAPPING

After curing is completed it's a good idea to wrap the soap to preserve both the appearance and the perfume. Use waxed paper, tissue or plastic wrap. Never use aluminium foil, as soap, because of its chemical composition, remains slightly alkaline.

MAKING SOAPS

There are several methods of making soap. Always remember that the contents of phase A are poured very slowly onto phase B, and that phase C is incorporated by thorough mixing when the soap is almost ready to pour. It's wise to make a test batch before embarking on the recipes below—you will gain confidence and expertise and avoid costly mistakes.

Ice cube trays can be used for small pretty-shaped soaps

Sponge bag, wire basket and shells from Linen and Lace of Balmain

Some beautiful ideas for wrapping and packaging home-made soaps for gifts

Basic Soap Method

PREPARATION

Read the cautions at the beginning of this chapter. Lay out all your equipment and ingredients in the order in which you will use them. Put on the apron and rubber gloves. Prepare the mould with either a damp cloth or petroleum jelly.

PHASE A
½ cup (125ml/4fl oz) cold distilled or purified
water or rainwater
25g (1oz) caustic soda

PHASE B
175ml (5½fl oz) melted clean tallow
25ml (1fl oz) oil

PHASE C
colouring and/or essential oils, additives

For phase A, have the water in a heatproof glass jug. Sprinkle in the caustic soda, stir until dissolved. Leave to cool to 33–34°C (91–93°F). Cooling is slow and can take up to an hour.

For phase B, have the melted tallow in a saucepan. Add the oil. Heat to 38–39°C (100–102°F).

When both phase mixtures reach the desired temperatures, pour the caustic mixture in a thin, slow stream into the tallow mixture, stirring constantly. This stirring should be done in a figure of eight and slowly. Stir…stir…stir… and stir some more, until a spoonful of the mixture holds a trail when drizzled on the surface of the soap. This can take from 10 to 60 minutes.

Crusty deposits (free caustic) which form on the sides of the bowl need to be scraped into the mixture. Make sure that you mix the scrapings in really well. The length of time taken to stir to the right consistency will depend largely on air temperature and the temperature of the mixture initially. Even if you are getting really bored and anxious you mustn't rush this stage or the soap won't set properly and might even separate into 2 layers.

Add any phase C ingredients, such as essential oil, talcum powder, almond meal etc. Incorporate really well but work quickly.

FINISHING

Pour the soap mix into the mould. Scrape any remaining in the bowl onto the mix using a spatula to smooth the surface of the bars. Put the mould in a warm place to harden the soap (an Esky is ideal but towels will serve).

When the soap is the consistency of hard butter it should be cut into bars (don't forget your gloves), replaced in the Esky and left for 24–48 hours.

The soap needs to mature in an airy place for 2–3 weeks before use. Stack so that as much surface as possible is exposed to the air. At the end of the curing time there may be a white film on the soap. This is free lye which may be scraped or washed off.

'Instant' Soap: Method 1

If the instructions above seem too time-consuming but you would like to incorporate some good things into commercial soap then you can start with either unperfumed soap (I use Velvet) or soap flakes (such as Lux).

The procedure is simple and the end product very good but it is an inexact way of adapting soap as the amount of fluid needed depends on the hardness of the base soap.

Grate the block of soap very finely—I use the stainless steel grater on my food processor.

Put the grated soap in the top of a non-aluminium double boiler and add triple strength infusion according to the individual recipes (in this chapter). Mix well. It's not necessary to stir constantly as the soap can take 1–3 hours to melt and rethicken.

When the mixture leaves a trail when trickled from the spoon it should be stirred until cooler and quite thick.

Any additives (e.g. essential oil, fine sand) may now be added, mixed in really well and the soap poured into moulds and left to set.

'Instant' Soap: Method 2

250g (8oz) grated soap or soap flakes
⅓ cup (80ml/2⅔fl oz) warm water or triple strength infusion
1 teaspoon essential oil
additives—colour, sand etc.

Combine the soap and water or triple strength infusion in a non-aluminium bowl and mix very well. Add the essential oil and any additives (e.g. fine sand, pumice, colouring) and mix until thoroughly combined.

Working quickly, knead all the ingredients together and mould into balls the size of golf balls or smooth the mixture into a mould.

If in a mould, stand until the soap is the consistency of hard butter, cut it into bars, then stand in an airy place until hardened.

If you make soap balls, stand them in an airy place until hardened.

Note: See the following page for step-by-step photographs

1. Finely grate the soap by hand or in the food processor

2. Measure and prepare all the other ingredients ready for mixing

3. Combine the soap and the remaining ingredients, mix thoroughly

4. Spread into a mould or shape into balls

Vegetarian Soap

This soap is for those who don't like using any animal products. It takes up to 2 hours to saponify and may take several weeks to harden. The resulting soap is fine and gentle but may not have as much lather as other soaps. Coconut essential oil is available as a flavouring for chocolate. It is not the same as coconut oil.

PHASE A
200ml (6½fl oz) water
20g (⅔oz) caustic soda
PHASE B
300g (10oz) coconut oil or Copha
100ml (3⅓fl oz) oil
PHASE C
3 teaspoons coconut essential oil
3 drops clove oil

For phase A, pour the water into a heatproof glass jug. Sprinkle the caustic soda over the water, stir until dissolved. Cool to 33–34°C (91–93°F).

Melt the phase B ingredients in a non-aluminium saucepan to 38–39°C (100–102°F).

When both phases are at the correct temperatures, pour the phase A mixture (caustic) slowly onto the phase B mixture (fats and oils). Stir constantly, using a wooden spoon.

Continue to stir, scraping crusty deposits from the side into the mixture, until the mixture forms a trail on the surface when drizzled from the wooden spoon.

Add the phase C ingredients, mix thoroughly and pour into prepared moulds.

Cucumber Soap

A pale green soap which smells and feels fresh and clean.

Note: To make the cucumber juice, blend ½ a chopped cucumber until pulped. Strain the juice and measure ⅓ cup (80ml/2⅔fl oz).

PHASE A
¾ cup (185ml/6fl oz) water
70g (2⅓oz) caustic soda
PHASE B
250g (8oz) tallow
50ml (1⅔fl oz) avocado oil
100ml (3⅓fl oz) coconut oil or Copha
PHASE C
1 teaspoon sage oil
1 teaspoon peppermint oil
½ teaspoon clove oil
⅓ cup (80ml/2⅔fl oz) cucumber juice (see note above)

For phase A, pour the water into a heatproof glass jug. Sprinkle the caustic soda over the water and stir until dissolved. Cool to 33–34°C (91–93°F).

Melt the phase B ingredients in a non-aluminium saucepan to 38–39°C (100–102°F).

When both phases are at the correct temperatures, pour the phase A mixture (caustic) slowly onto the phase B mixture (fats and oils). Stir constantly, using a wooden spoon. Continue to stir, scraping crusty deposits from the side into the mixture, until the mixture forms a trail on the surface when drizzled from the spoon.

Add the phase C ingredients, mix thoroughly and pour into prepared moulds.

Sesame and Almond Soap

This is a lovely soap. It has a good lather, feels very softening and, at the same time, it has a very gentle, mildly abrasive action which removes dead surface skin.

PHASE A
200ml (6½fl oz) water
70g (2⅓oz) caustic soda
PHASE B
200g (6½oz) tallow
50ml (1⅔fl oz) almond oil
100ml (3⅓fl oz) coconut oil or Copha
50ml (1⅔fl oz) sesame oil
PHASE C
20g (⅔oz) ground almonds
1 teaspoon rose geranium oil
1 teaspoon lavender oil
½ teaspoon clove oil

For phase A, pour the water into a heatproof glass jug. Sprinkle the caustic soda over the water, stir until dissolved. Cool to 33–34°C (91–93°F).

Melt the phase B ingredients in a non-aluminium saucepan to 38–39°C (100–102°F).

When both phases are at the correct temperatures, pour the phase A mixture (caustic) slowly onto the phase B mixture (fats and oils). Stir constantly using a wooden spoon. Continue to stir, scraping crusty deposits from the side into the mixture, until the mixture forms a trail on the surface when drizzled from the spoon.

Add the phase C ingredients, mix thoroughly and pour into prepared moulds.

Caraway Soap

One of my favourite soaps. It feels soft and gentle and smells spicy and delicious. Crush the caraway seeds really well before making the infusion and strain through coffee filter paper. If you can make the infusion the day before and leave it to infuse overnight it will be much improved.

PHASE A
100ml (3⅓fl oz) water
70g (2⅓oz) caustic soda
PHASE B
300g (approx 10oz) tallow
50ml (1⅔fl oz) olive oil
50ml (1⅔fl oz) coconut oil or Copha
PHASE C
150ml (5fl oz) triple strength caraway infusion
3 teaspoons powdered caraway
1½ teaspoons caraway oil
½ teaspoon orange oil
25 drops sandalwood oil

For phase A, pour the water into a heatproof glass jug. Sprinkle the caustic soda over the water, stir until dissolved. Cool to 33–34°C (91–93°F).

Melt the phase B ingredients in a non-aluminium saucepan to 38–39°C (100–102°F).

When both phases are at the correct temperatures, pour the phase A mixture (caustic) slowly onto the phase B mixture (fats and oils). Stir constantly using a wooden spoon. Continue to stir, scraping crusty deposits from the side into the mixture, until the mixture forms a trail on the surface when drizzled from the spoon.

Add the phase C ingredients, mix thoroughly and pour into prepared moulds.

Egg and Chamomile Soap

Gentle enough for baby skin. Both egg and chamomile are renowned for their beneficial properties. Leave to mature for at least 6 weeks.

PHASE A

1 cup (250ml/8fl oz) water

70g (2⅓oz) caustic soda

PHASE B

250g (8oz) tallow

50ml (1⅔fl oz) coconut oil or Copha

PHASE C

2 egg yolks

⅓ cup (80ml/2⅔fl oz) olive oil

1 teaspoon runny honey

1 teaspoon chamomile oil

1 teaspoon sandalwood oil

For phase A, pour the water into a heatproof glass jug. Sprinkle the caustic soda over the water, stir until dissolved. Cool to 33–34°C (91–93°F).

Melt the phase B ingredients in a non-aluminium saucepan to 38–39°C (100–102°F).

When both phases are at the correct temperatures, pour the phase A mixture (caustic) slowly onto the phase B mixture (fats and oils). Stir constantly using a wooden spoon. Continue to stir, scraping crusty deposits from the side into the mixture, until the mixture forms a trail on the surface when drizzled from the spoon.

Add the phase C ingredients, mix thoroughly and pour into prepared moulds.

Medicated Soap for Troubled Skins

This is a useful soap for spotty or blemished skins.

PHASE A

1 cup (250ml/8fl oz) distilled or purified water or rainwater

70g (2⅓oz) caustic soda

PHASE B

300g (10oz) tallow

100g (3⅓oz) coconut oil or Copha

PHASE C

¼ cup (30g/1oz) ground oats

2 teaspoons tea tree oil

For phase A, pour the water into a heatproof glass jug. Sprinkle the caustic soda over the water, stir until dissolved. Cool to 33–34°C (91–93°F).

Melt the phase B ingredients in a non-aluminium saucepan to 38–39°C (100–102°F).

When both phases are at the correct temperatures, pour the phase A mixture (caustic) slowly onto the phase B mixture (fats and oils). Stir constantly using a wooden spoon. Continue to stir, scraping crusty deposits from the side into the mixture, until the mixture forms a trail on the surface when drizzled from the spoon.

Add the phase C ingredients, mix thoroughly and pour into prepared moulds.

Herb Soap

You can add gravy browning for a rich brown.

PHASE A

½ cup (125ml/4fl oz) water

70g (2⅓oz) caustic soda

PHASE B

200g (6½oz) tallow

100ml (3⅓fl oz) elderflower oil (see Making a Herb Oil Base in Chapter One)

100ml (3⅓fl oz) coconut oil or Copha

PHASE C

½ cup (125ml/4fl oz) elderflower infusion

¼ cup (30g/1oz) talcum powder

2 teaspoons lavender oil

½ teaspoon tincture of benzoin

2 teaspoons melted lanolin

For phase A, pour the water into a heatproof glass jug. Sprinkle the caustic soda over the water, stir until dissolved. Cool to 33–34°C (91–93°F).

Melt the phase B ingredients in a non-aluminium saucepan to 38–39°C (100–102°F).

When both phases are at the correct temperatures, pour the phase A mixture (caustic) slowly onto the phase B mixture (fats and oils). Stir constantly using a wooden spoon. Continue to stir, scraping crusty deposits from the side into the mixture, until the mixture forms a trail on the surface when drizzled from the spoon.

Add the phase C ingredients, mix thoroughly and pour into prepared moulds.

Soap for 'Him'

I would hate to have an accusation of 'sexism' levelled at me but I think that some soaps smell masculine and others feminine. The following soap is perfumed with sandalwood, cedarwood and bergamot—very suitable for the blokes but if you are a girl and you like it then use it!

PHASE A
200ml (6½fl oz) water
70g (2⅓oz) caustic soda
PHASE B
250g (8oz) tallow
100ml (3⅓fl oz) coconut oil or Copha
PHASE C
1 teaspoon sandalwood oil
1 teaspoon cedarwood oil
½ teaspoon bergamot oil
3 teaspoons paprika mixed with
50ml (1⅔fl oz) sesame oil

For phase A, pour the water into a heatproof glass jug. Sprinkle the caustic soda over the water, stir until dissolved. Cool to 33–34°C (91–93°F).

Melt the phase B ingredients in a non-aluminium saucepan to 38–39°C (100–102°F).

When both phases are at the correct temperatures, pour the phase A mixture (caustic) slowly onto the phase B mixture (fats and oils). Stir constantly using a wooden spoon. Continue to stir, scraping crusty deposits from the side into the mixture, until the mixture forms a trail on the surface when drizzled from the spoon.

Add the phase C ingredients, mix thoroughly and pour into prepared moulds.

Spicy Boys

PHASE A
250g (8oz) grated soap or soap flakes
½ cup (125ml/4fl oz) warm water
PHASE B
¼ cup (30g/1oz) ground rolled oats
PHASE C
1 drop nutmeg oil
3 drops pine oil
4 drops lemon oil
2 drops sandalwood oil

Melt the phase A ingredients together in a double boiler. This may take some time. Add the phase B ingredient, stir well to incorporate. Add the phase C ingredients and mix well. Either press into moulds or cool until mouldable and the mixture can be formed into balls.

Leave in an airy place to harden.

Anti-Mossie Soap

If mosquitoes love to bite you then this soap will provide partial protection. This soap is best made by the 'double batching' method (see Perfuming Soap early in this chapter) in order to keep the maximum benefits from the essential oils, or make it using the method given, although it will not be as protective.

PHASE A
200ml (6½fl oz) water
70g (2⅓oz) caustic soda
PHASE B
200g (6½oz) tallow
50ml (1⅔fl oz) olive oil
100ml (3⅓fl oz) coconut oil or Copha
PHASE C
1 teaspoon citronella oil
1 teaspoon lavender oil
½ teaspoon eucalyptus oil

For phase A, pour the water into a heatproof glass jug. Sprinkle the caustic soda over the water, stir until dissolved. Cool to 33–34°C (91–93°F).

Melt the phase B ingredients in a non-aluminium saucepan to 38–39°C (100–102°F).

When both phases are at the correct temperatures, pour the phase A mixture (caustic) slowly onto the phase B mixture (fats and oils). Stir constantly using a wooden spoon. Continue to stir, scraping crusty deposits from the side into the mixture, until the mixture forms a trail on the surface when drizzled from the spoon.

Add the phase C ingredients, mix thoroughly and pour into prepared moulds.

Making Egg and Chamomile Soap

Cream Soap

This soap has little lather but is so gentle on your skin that you will overlook the lack of froth. A good face or body cream or any of the 'oil-in-water' moisture cream recipes in this book will be suitable. Don't try adding the 'water-in-oil' emulsions as the effect won't be the same.

PHASE A
250g (8oz) finely grated soap or soap flakes
½ cup (125ml/4fl oz) warm water
PHASE B
60g (2oz) moisture cream
PHASE C
6 drops lavender oil
3 drops geranium oil
2 drops rosemary oil

Melt the phase A ingredients together in a double boiler. This may take some time. Add the phase B ingredient and stir well to incorporate. Add the phase C ingredients and mix well. Either press into moulds or cool until mouldable and the mixture can be formed into balls.

Leave in an airy place to harden.

QUICK SOAPS

The following recipes are made from ready-made soap, either soapflakes (e.g. 'Lux') or unperfumed, grated soap (e.g. 'Velvet'). This is a quick and efficient way of making soap. It's easiest to mould this soap into balls as it can't easily be made into blocks.

Hand Cleanser

PHASE A
250g (8oz) grated soap or soap flakes
¾ cup (185ml/6fl oz) triple strength
elderflower infusion
PHASE B
1 teaspoon sesame oil
2 tablespoons olive oil
1 tablespoon elderflower oil (see Making a Herb
Oil Base in Chapter One)

PHASE C
200g (6½oz) powdered pumice or fine sand
1 teaspoon lemon oil
1 teaspoon sandalwood oil

Melt the phase A ingredients together in a double boiler. This may take some time. Add the phase B ingredients and stir well to incorporate.

Add the phase C ingredients, mix well and either press into prepared moulds or cool until mouldable and the mixture can be formed into balls. Leave in an airy place to harden.

Lettuce and Parsley Soap

Both these ingredients are good for your skin. The soap is a pretty, green colour and smells lovely and fresh.

PHASE A
250g (8oz) grated soap or soap flakes
½ cup (125ml/4fl oz) warm lettuce and
parsley water
PHASE B
30g (1oz) melted lanolin
PHASE C
1 teaspoon peppermint oil
½ teaspoon lemon oil

Melt the phase A ingredients together in a double boiler. This may take some time. Add the phase B ingredient, stir well to incorporate. Add the phase C ingredients and mix well. Either press into moulds or cool until mouldable and the mixture can be formed into balls.

Leave in an airy place to harden.

Note: To make the lettuce and parsley water: Blend (in a food processor) a handful of parsley and 4–6 dark green lettuce leaves, with about 1 tablespoon water and 1 tablespoon vodka. Strain through cheesecloth and squeeze to get every drop of juice. Make up to ½ cup (125ml/4fl oz) with purified or distilled water or rainwater.

Clockwise from top: Lettuce and Parsley Soap, Spicy Boys, Herb Soap, Vegetarian Soap

Bath rack and silver shell soap dish from Linen and Lace of Balmain; bath brushes from Crabtree & Evelyn; soaps from Nirala

AROMATHERAPY AND PERFUMES

Our sense of smell is the most evocative sense we possess as it is

connected to the part of the brain responsible for memory. Which of us

is not transported back to other places, other days, by a sudden waft

of perfume? My strongest memories are evoked by the smells of

old-fashioned carnations, mandarins, freshly

percolated coffee, and shoe polish!

Tassle from Linen and Lace of Balmain

*Aromatherapy has a special
place in every situation*

THE 'PECULIAR CHARMERS'

Thou perceivest the Flowers put forth their
precious odours;
And none can tell how from so small a centre
comes such sweet.
—WILLIAM BLAKE (1757–1827)

This chapter is an introduction to the art of aromatherapy and perfumery. My dictionary describes aroma as 'spicy, fragrant; having peculiar charm'—I like the last one particularly!

These days our sense of smell is assaulted by synthetic perfumes and chemicals—a visit to the supermarket can be a nightmare to a sensitive nose as it absorbs the synthetic perfumes from soaps, cleaning agents and insecticides. We can avoid these unpleasant smells in our homes by making our own products and using essential oils to enhance and perfume them.

THE USE OF AROMATICS AND ESSENTIAL OILS

The use of essential oil by plants has not yet been understood. Some plants, such as citrus fruits, contain oil in profusion, others, such as jasmine contain little oil but this small amount is incredibly strongly scented. Other plants appear to contain no oil at all. There are indications that oil extraction from plants has been carried out since 3000 BC and records show that the oils were used for religious ceremonies, being used as oils for anointing, incense for burning and waters for washing both priests and altars; two of the gifts brought to Jesus by the wise men were the exquisitely perfumed resins frankincense and myrrh. Three thousand years ago aromatics were being used in China, India and Egypt and were a large part of their trade; ships sailed through perilous waters carrying their precious and luxurious cargoes among which were spices, scented woods, gums, resins and camphor:

Quinquereme of Nineveh from distant Ophir
Rowing home to haven in sunny Palestine,
With a cargo of ivory, and apes
and peacocks,
Sandalwood, cedarwood, and
sweet white wine.
—JOHN MASEFIELD (1878–1967)

Many books suggest that the main use (apart from religious ceremonies) of the crudely extracted oils from aromatic botanicals was to mask and disguise the smells of dirty places and people. I feel that this is doing a disservice to the intelligence of the people who used the herbs and oils. If we examine the biblical references we discover that the herbs and oils mentioned all had strongly therapeutic actions—surely not an accident.

Essential oils are volatile compounds that occur naturally in plants. In some cases the oil is excreted, giving the plant a characteristic scent which attracts insects; in others the oil isn't apparent unless the plant is crushed or dried (the root of valerian being an example). Some oils are not apparent until incisions are made in the bark to release the resin or gum of the plant and many of these have no perfume until they are dried.

Essential oils have been variously described as the 'life force' or 'essence' of plants. The essential oil is contained in minuscule quantities in most plants; consequently many finished oils are very expensive.

The essence or essential oil of plants is found in leaves (such as eucalyptus), petals (rose), bark (sandalwood), resins (myrrh), roots (calamus), rind (citrus fruits) and seeds (caraway).

The word 'oil' causes some confusion as people tend to think of these essences as being the same as olive, safflower and other 'fixed' oils. Essential oils are non-oily and, unlike the fixed oils, they evaporate when exposed to air.

The term 'aromatherapy' was first used in the 1920s by René Maurice Gattefosse, a French chemist who used the term to describe 'a therapy using aromatics'. One account states that Gattefosse burnt his hand and thrust it into the nearest liquid to quell the pain; the liquid happened to be a tub of lavender oil which not only eased the pain but caused the burn to heal very quickly.

The word 'aromatherapy' implies that the cure or treatment lies in the inhalation of the aroma (perfume) of the plant extract being used. Whilst this is true, it is only part of the story. These precious essences are composed of molecules small enough to penetrate the skin and enter the blood stream and so may be employed in many ways:

➤ incorporating with carrier oils to make massage oils
➤ adding to water to use as fomentations and compresses
➤ adding in minute quantities to baths
➤ adding to alcohol to make toilet waters and perfumes
➤ incorporating with any carrier to make insect repellents
➤ incorporating in cosmetic creams and healing ointments
➤ using in shampoos, conditioners and hair tonics
➤ strengthening the perfume of potpourris
➤ adding antibacterial qualities to room freshener sprays
➤ using in preparations for pets, to heal skin conditions and repel fleas
➤ adding to floor and furniture cleaners

CAUTIONS

Some of the essences are very toxic and should only be used internally on the advice of a qualified aromatherapist or naturopath. As little as $\frac{1}{2}$ teaspoon of eucalyptus oil taken internally has proved fatal.

All essential oils should be kept well out of the reach of children as most would prove lethal if drunk—even in small quantities.

It is essential that you read the following information carefully noting the cautions, as some oils are toxic in large quantities and others must be avoided in some conditions.

Most of the oils should be combined with a 'carrier' (or 'base') oil such as olive or sweet almond oil before using externally as they are too strong to use alone. The total amount of all essential oils used (either singly or combined with other ingredients) in a blend should never exceed 3% of the total amount and some oils should be used in far smaller amounts. See Blending and Diluting the Oils in this chapter.

It's imperative to use only the best essential oils available; synthetics and compounded oils don't have the healing properties of the 'real thing' and could be dangerous if taken internally.

Many oils are labelled as 'fragrant oil', 'compounded oil', 'perfume oil'. These descriptions mean that the oil is synthetic, or blended with either paraffin oil or a carrier oil. Check with the retailer that the oil labelled '100% pure, natural, essential oil' is in fact what it purports to be; if in doubt, wait until you find a reliable source.

Another check is cost. If oils such as rose, jasmine or neroli (to mention but a few) are roughly the same price as the more common lavender, rosemary and peppermint, then they are almost certainly not the real thing.

SPECIFIC CAUTIONS

SITUATION OR EFFECT	OILS TO AVOID
*ALLERGIC REACTIONS	Aniseed, bay, citronella, clove, jasmine
EPILEPSY	Fennel, hyssop, rosemary.
PREGNANCY	Basil, cedarwood, citronella, clary sage, fennel, hyssop, juniper, marjoram, myrrh, nutmeg, peppermint, rosemary, sage, thyme
EXTRA POWERFUL	Thyme and peppermint oil should never exceed 0.5–1%
NARCOTIC	Aniseed, clary sage, coriander, fennel, nutmeg
**PHOTOTOXICITY	Bergamot, lemon, lime, orange

NOTE

* ALLERGIC REACTION	These oils may cause an allergic reaction in sensitive individuals.
** PHOTOTOXIC	An oil which may cause pigmentation if applied to skin which will be exposed to the sun.

METHODS OF EXTRACTION

Most commercial extraction such as distillation and solvent extraction requires the use of sophisticated equipment and methods which are largely beyond the scope of the home user.

There are three methods however which may be used at home with varying degrees of success depending on the quality and quantity of the herb used and the patience and diligence of the herb collector!

ENFLEURAGE

A time-honoured method of recovering essential oil from petals which retain their perfume for some time after collection (such as tuberose, rose and jasmine) is called 'enfleurage'. This is becoming a dying art as the cost of skilled labour becomes prohibitive for commercial oil producers. This method is easy (if time-consuming) to do at home:

Enfleurage Method

1 Spread a thin layer of pure lard or hardened vegetable fat (not margarine) on a glass or enamel sheet.

2 Press a single layer of heavily perfumed fresh flower petals onto the fat. Lay another sheet of glass on top. Leave for 24 hours. Pick the petals off the fat and replace with more.

3 Repeat the above process for 7–21 days or until the perfume is as strong as you desire.

4 Pick off the petals and scrape the fat into a bowl. Cover the bowl and place into a pan of hot water to melt the fat. Don't overheat or the oil will evaporate.

5 Add a few drops of a fixative oil such as sandalwood, pour the melted fat into little pots and put lids on at once.

The resulting scented fat is called a sachet or cream perfume and may be used in the same way as liquid perfume. If you prefer a liquid cologne/toilet water, you can stop the above after stage 3 and proceed as follows:

4 Pick off the petals and either scrape the fat into a jar or, if hard, chop into walnut-sized pieces.

5 Cover with vodka or other high-proof alcohol which has little or no smell.

6 Cover with a leakproof lid and store in a dark place for 3–4 weeks, shaking daily.

7 Strain or skim the fat from the alcohol, add a few drops of one of the fixative oils to the alcohol and pour into small, well-stoppered bottles. Now you have genuine home-made cologne.

If, after removing the fat (stage 7), the alcohol is evaporated off in a double boiler over a very gentle heat, you will be left with pure essential oil. The amount however will be minuscule and there is always a danger of overheating and evaporating the oil along with the alcohol.

MACERATION

If you have masses of perfumed petals you can use the following method to make a deliciously scented oil. The petals don't have to be from the same type of flower as a mixed perfume blend can be very pleasant.

The method is very simple but a steady, very gentle source of heat is essential. I put the jar on top of the refrigerator, towards the back where the rising heat from the coils remains gentle and constant.

Maceration Method

Quarter fill a jar with cotton wool balls. Cover them with an unscented oil such as sweet almond or grapeseed. Pack the jar with fresh, slightly crushed, heavily scented petals. Cover with a tightly fitting lid and leave in a constantly warm place for 2 days.

Take out the petals and replace with fresh ones. Repeat these procedures for up to a month.

Squeeze the cotton wool balls to extract as much perfume oil as possible.

EXPRESSION

The oil in citrus plants is contained in glands in the outer skin. Before machines were invented to replace humans, the skins of the citrus were squeezed by hand until the glands burst, the droplets being collected in sponges which were then squeezed to collect the oil in containers.

This squeezing method can be used at home. Collect the droplets with a small cosmetic sponge or cotton wool balls, or wrap a small piece of cheesecloth around the fruit. If the amount of oil collected is too small to squeeze out, the sponge or ball can be dropped into a little vodka or almond oil, left overnight and then squeezed out, leaving the essential oil in the alcohol or carrier oil. This is a good way of making full use of skins which would otherwise be wasted.

BLENDING AND DILUTING THE OILS

For ease of measuring and for safety's sake, I would strongly advise you to buy accurate measurers.

A pharmacist will usually be able to supply, or tell you where to obtain, a dropper which is marked in amounts up to 1ml (18–20 drops) and glass or plastic (not as good) beakers or hypodermic syringes which will measure amounts from 1ml (18–20 drops) upwards.

A set of metric measuring spoons is more accurate than regular household spoons, but still not as good as those made to pharmaceutical or laboratory standards.

> 18–20 drops = 1ml = 1 marked dropper
> 90–100 drops = 5ml = 1 metric teaspoon
> 20ml = 1 metric tablespoon

In any sized bottle the main content will be a carrier such as oil, vinegar or alcohol in which to dilute the essential oils. (A 'carrier oil' is also known as a 'base oil'.) The following chart gives the amounts of essential oils to add in order to achieve 1%, 2% or 3% dilution.

BLENDING CHART

100ml ($3\frac{1}{2}$fl oz) bottle
18–20 drops = 1ml in 100ml ($3\frac{1}{3}$fl oz) bottle = approx 1%
30–40 drops = 2ml in 100ml ($3\frac{1}{3}$fl oz) bottle = approx 2%
54–60 drops = 3ml in 100ml ($3\frac{1}{3}$fl oz) bottle = approx 3%

50ml ($1\frac{2}{3}$fl oz) bottle
9–10 drops = 0.5ml in 50ml ($1\frac{2}{3}$fl oz) bottle = approx 1%
18–20 drops = 1ml in 50ml ($1\frac{2}{3}$fl oz) bottle = approx 2%
27–30 drops = 1.5ml in 50ml ($1\frac{2}{3}$fl oz) bottle = approx 3%

10ml ($\frac{1}{3}$fl oz) bottle
2 drops in 10ml ($\frac{1}{3}$fl oz) bottle = approx 1%
4 drops in 10ml ($\frac{1}{3}$fl oz) bottle = approx 2%
6 drops in 10ml ($\frac{1}{3}$fl oz) bottle = approx 3%

BLENDING GUIDE

The following list gives a general idea of the amounts to use, bearing in mind the above comments. Individual recipes may specify more or less.

Massage oils   2–2.5%

Face oils   1–1.5%

Fomentations and compresses   10 drops in 100ml ($3\frac{1}{3}$fl oz)

Ointments   3%

Creams and lotions   1–1.5%

Baths   10 drops maximum. Swish the water really well to disperse the essential oil or add the essential oil to 1 tablespoon olive oil, vodka or full-cream milk and pour it into the bath. Swish well.

Toilet waters/perfumes   Varies. See pertinent recipes.

Insect repellent rubs   2–2.5%

Room sprays, all types   1 teaspoon in 50ml ($1\frac{2}{3}$fl oz) alcohol. Dissolve and add 1 cup (250ml/8fl oz) purified water.

Shampoos and conditioners   1–1.5%

Potpourris   Varies. See pertinent recipes.

Pet shampoo   1 drop in shampoo; 1 more in rinsing water.

Floor and furniture cleaners   2% or whatever smells good!

DIRECTORY OF ESSENTIAL OILS

This section contains reference lists of some of the main properties and uses of essential oils. There are many more which you will discover as your interest in them grows.

By cross-matching these lists you will be able to create oil blends which reflect your personality and are both practical and aesthetic. Experiment with tiny amounts until you are satisfied, as the oils are too precious to waste.

A FEW FAVOURITE OILS

I have a great affection for most of the essential oils but there are a few to which I find myself particularly drawn. By accident or subconscious design these few favourites cover almost every situation which arises. You will discover your own favourites as you use and learn more about the oils, but it is initially the part of your brain responsible for memory that will determine the oils to which you will first be attracted.

There will be oils which have an impressive list of uses but which have no appeal to you—this may be because the odour is subconsciously connected to an unpleasant incident or person in your childhood. I feel that there is little value to be gained from the use of an oil which is unpleasant (for whatever reason) to you.

There are a couple of oils which, while they have many valuable properties are so unappealing to me that I rarely, if ever, use them. One of the oils which I find quite repugnant is patchouli. It makes me think of the type of 'hippie' in the 60s who rarely or never washed their bodies (we weren't all like that) and tried (and failed) to cover their smell with this earthy and deep fragrance. Young friends who don't remember this colourful decade can't understand my reluctance to use this oil, as to them, it is romantic, sensual and exotic.

Another observation I would make is that the oils to which we are most drawn are often the ones which are most beneficial to us personally. I believe that the body has its own 'mind' and recognises what it needs. If you particularly like the perfume of an oil, study the benefits to be obtained from that oil and it is likely that you will find they are the ones which you need physically, emotionally or mentally at the time.

The following oils are my current favourites. Some (like lavender and rosemary) have been on the list since my childhood and are part of my 'security blanket', all have been in favour for many years but, who knows, I may add or subtract an oil in the future as my needs change. The list contains my reason as to why I use these particular oils but I wouldn't suggest that it be followed slavishly or have it assumed that these are the oils on which you will base you own favourite selection. Your choices will be determined by your age, the ages of your family and your lifestyle.

Try as many oils as you can before you buy them. Buy only the best; the most authentic and pure. Buy only one oil at a time, learn and absorb its magic and let it become a trusted friend before your next step in this new adventure.

Above all—enjoy!

GRAPEFRUIT

My morning saviour is grapefruit oil. It doesn't possess as many properties as many other oils but my affection stems from the fact that the irresistible sweet, sharp and refreshing smell helps me to get going in the morning when I am definitely not at my best. A bath or shower oil and body lotion containing this oil will not only uplift your spirits but will also stimulate the lymphatic system, act as a tonic to the liver and help to get rid of cellulite by its effect on water retention.

This oil is a boon to travellers as it seems to help the body to avoid exhaustion and jet lag. Use it to lift your spirits and energy when life feels dull and flat.

LAVENDER

Lavender would have to be my number one favourite and the one oil which I carry everywhere I go; it seems to have been part of my life since childhood. Many people associate lavender with lace, old ladies, garden hedges and potpourris without realising the therapeutic potential hidden in this floral, freshly sweet smelling oil which is so gentle that it is suitable for all age groups.

It may be used undiluted but as a rule it is more economical and useful if 4ml (80 drops) of lavender oil are put into a 25ml (1fl oz) bottle which is then filled with almond oil. This small bottle can be carried in the pocket or handbag and the oil used to repel insects or ease their bites; to lessen stress and stress headaches; as a rub for sprains or strains; a remedy to ease sunburn (which shouldn't happen!) and minor burns and scalds; to massage on pulse points or sniff from the bottle to create an atmosphere of calm and restore mental and emotional order; used on scratches, grazes, sores and other wounds to help prevent sepsis and accelerate healing.

GERANIUM

When I was young and impressionable my most admired fictional heroine used only geranium oil as her scent, naturally I felt that some of her glamour and style would become mine if I too wore the same perfume!

I've grown up a bit since those days but this oil still features in my 'top oils' as over the years I became more and more aware of its benefits to women of all ages but particularly during menopause. It works profoundly on the emotions, lifting the spirits and alleviating stress; acts as a hormonal regulator and has a tonic action on the lymphatic system, the liver and kidneys.

Geranium oil and chamomile oil mixed with a carrier oil make the finest treatment for sore, lumpy or otherwise troubled breasts. These are just a few of the benefits of this oil and as a bonus—it smells wonderful.

TEA TREE

Tea tree must have an important place in this chat about favourite oils, as it is antibacterial, antifungal and antiviral making it useful for a wide range of problems such as athlete's foot, gum problems and mouth ulcers, skin infections, acne and sunburn. This makes it a good choice for the first aid box.

Tea tree oil is very safe to use and apart from lavender is the only oil which can be used neat in an emergency. I prefer to dilute it as it works well and costs less. I use the same dilution as for lavender oil.

ROSEMARY

No list of the important oils would be complete without the inclusion of rosemary. Known as the Herb of Remembrance, it has both romantic and practical association. It is a well known mental stimulant—very useful for students or others who use their brains very intensively.

Rosemary is a highly stimulating oil and as such, is useful for correcting low blood pressure and strengthening weak hearts; giving strength and tone to overworked muscles; easing headaches and reducing the levels of stress; boosting the action of the entire digestive system; tightening the skin tissue and encouraging hair growth. It's strengthening for the immune system.

PALMAROSA

Many people are surprised at my inclusion of palmarosa in my list of favourite oils as it is one of the less well known oils. The odour of this lovely oil is warm, sweet/dry and rosy, it 'holds' other perfumes really well in blends and is one of the few oils which can be used in home-made soap without completely losing its perfume.

It is my preferred skin oil as it stimulates cell regeneration, regulates sebum production, moisturises and generally helps to retard wrinkles.

Palmarosa refreshes and uplifts the emotions, eases nervous exhaustion and is useful during stressful situations.

Rose oil is also a very popular essential oil

Flowers by Lisa Milasas

PEPPERMINT

Peppermint is the only oil that I feel I need to use internally. One drop mixed with a little honey, dissolved into a glass of warm water and sipped has an almost instantaneous effect on travel nausea or the indigestion caused by eating too much or eating rich foods. A small flask containing this mixture can prevent a lot of misery if you are a poor traveller. This same mixture will often ease a 'digestive' headache or stomach cramps. It should not be used in pregnancy but spearmint may be substituted to alleviate morning sickness.

Peppermint oil needs to be treated with some respect and the amount used in massage oils and other external treatments should never exceed 1% which is about 18–20 drops in 80 drops of oil, alcohol, water or other carrier.

SANDALWOOD

This magical and beautiful oil is one of the oldest known perfumes. Records going back as far as 4000 years make mention of its use for embalming, perfumery, making incense and healing many illnesses. It blends wonderfully with almost all other oils and acts as a rich, exotic base note and fixative in perfumes.

Sandalwood reaches deep into the recesses and deep, secret parts of our mind and psyche. I carry this oil because it makes me feel calm, tranquil and meditative even during the most stressful times. I also use it in most of my personal perfume blends and would include it in blends for easing problems of the urinary, digestive and respiratory systems.

CLASSIFICATION BY 'NOTES'

Essential oils are classified as 'top', 'middle' and 'base' notes.

TOP NOTES
Top notes are the most fleeting, the sharpest, the clearest and most uplifting. They are the violins of the perfume orchestra; they are the first impression to the nose, and the aroma (if no fixative is used) lasts for 24 hours or much less.

MIDDLE NOTES
Middle notes are the violas—they give substance to the perfume and are more stable, soft and 'round'. If unfixed, the scent lasts for up to three days.

BASE NOTES
Base notes are strong, intense and deep like the rich, deep sounds of the cello. They have sedating and relaxing qualities, the lowest volatility and therefore the longest-lasting perfume, which makes them ideal as fixatives.

In order to create a long-lasting, balanced perfume it's essential to understand and include oils with top, middle and base notes. Don't let the following information make you feel nervous or insecure. You can create simple perfumes at first and as you become more familiar and confident with the oils your sense of adventure will take over—you may end up creating a challenge to the perfume houses of Paris!

CLASSIFICATION
OF ESSENTIAL OILS BY NOTES

TOP NOTES	TOP TO MIDDLE NOTES	MIDDLE NOTES	MIDDLE TO BASE NOTES	BASE NOTES
OIL	OIL	OIL	OIL	OIL
basil	aniseed	black pepper	cypress	benzoin
bay	clary sage	chamomile	frankincense	cedarwood
bergamot	fennel	citronella	jasmine	cinnamon
caraway	mandarin	clove	neroli	clove
cardamom	thyme	geranium	rose	myrrh
citronella	petitgrain	hyssop	ylang-ylang	patchouli
coriander		pine		sandalwood
dill		juniper		vetiver
eucalyptus		lavender		
ginger		marjoram		
grapefruit		melissa		
lemon		nutmeg		
lemon grass		rosemary		
lime		rosewood		
niaouli		thyme		
nutmeg				
orange				
palmarosa				
peppermint				
spearmint				
tea tree				

GOOD FRIEND BLENDS

This is a list of essential oils and other oils with which they blend.
Before you experiment with oil blending you would be advised to read the foregoing
section on 'Notes'. Even though the following lists contain oils which are happy together
you could end up with a scent which is very unbalanced unless you include top, middle
and base notes in your blend.

OIL	BLENDS WITH
BASIL	Bergamot, black pepper, clary sage, geranium, hyssop, lavender, lemon grass, marjoram, melissa, neroli, sandalwood
BENZOIN	Bergamot, cypress, eucalyptus, frankincense, juniper, lavender, lemon, myrrh, orange, petitgrain, rose, sandalwood
BERGAMOT	Basil, benzoin, chamomile, cypress, eucalyptus, geranium, juniper, jasmine, lavender, lemon, marjoram, neroli, palmarosa, patchouli, ylang-ylang
BLACK PEPPER	Basil, bergamot, cypress, frankincense, geranium, grapefruit, lemon, palmarosa, rosemary, sandalwood, ylang-ylang
CEDARWOOD	Benzoin, bergamot, cinnamon, cypress, frankincense, jasmine, juniper, lavender, lemon, neroli, rose, rosemary
CHAMOMILE	Benzoin, bergamot, geranium, jasmine, lavender, lemon, marjoram, neroli, palmarosa, patchouli, rose, ylang-ylang
CINNAMON	Benzoin, clove, frankincense, ginger, grapefruit, lavender, orange, pine, rosemary, thyme
CLARY SAGE	Basil, bergamot, cedarwood, cypress, frankincense, geranium, grapefruit, jasmine, juniper, lavender, sandalwood
CLOVE	Basil, benzoin, black pepper, cinnamon, grapefruit, lemon, nutmeg, orange, peppermint, rosemary
CORIANDER	Bergamot, black pepper, cinnamon, cypress, geranium
CYPRESS	Benzoin, bergamot, clary sage, juniper, lavender, lemon, orange, pine, rosemary, sandalwood
EUCALYPTUS	Benzoin, bergamot, coriander, juniper, lavender, lemon, lemon grass, melissa, pine, thyme

FENNEL	Basil, geranium, lavender, lemon, rose, rosemary, sandalwood	**LEMON**	Benzoin, bergamot, chamomile, eucalyptus, fennel, frankincense, ginger, juniper, lavender, neroli, rose, sandalwood, ylang-ylang
FRANKINCENSE	Benzoin, black pepper, geranium, grapefruit, lavender, orange, melissa, patchouli, pine, sandalwood	**LEMON GRASS**	Basil, cedarwood, coriander, geranium, jasmine, lavender, neroli, palmarosa, rosemary, tea tree
GERANIUM	Basil, bergamot, cedarwood, clary sage, grapefruit, jasmine, lavender, lime, neroli, orange, petitgrain, rose, rosemary, sandalwood	**LIME**	Bergamot, geranium, lavender, neroli, nutmeg, palmarosa, rose, ylang-ylang
GINGER	All spice oils, eucalyptus, frankincense, geranium, lemon, lime, orange, rosemary, spearmint	**MANDARIN**	Basil, bergamot, black pepper, coriander, chamomile, grapefruit, lavender, lemon, lime, marjoram, neroli, palmarosa, petitgrain, rose
GRAPEFRUIT	Basil, bergamot, cedarwood, chamomile, frankincense, geranium, jasmine, lavender, palmarosa, rose, rosewood, ylang-ylang	**MARJORAM**	Basil, bergamot, cedarwood, chamomile, cypress, lavender, mandarin, marjoram, orange, nutmeg, rosemary, rosewood, ylang-ylang
HYSSOP	Basil, fennel, lavender, melissa, orange, rosemary, mandarin	**MELISSA**	Basil, chamomile, frankincense, geranium, ginger, jasmine, juniper, lavender, marjoram, neroli, rose, rosemary, ylang-ylang
JASMINE	Bergamot, frankincense, geranium, orange, mandarin, melissa, neroli, palmarosa, rose, rosewood, sandalwood	**MYRRH**	Benzoin, clove, frankincense, lavender, patchouli, sandalwood
JUNIPER	Benzoin, bergamot, cypress, frankincense, geranium, grapefruit, orange, lemon grass, lime, melissa, rosemary, sandalwood	**NEROLI**	Basil, benzoin, bergamot, coriander, geranium, jasmine, lavender, lemon, lime, orange, palmarosa, petitgrain, rose, rosemary, sandalwood, ylang-ylang
LAVENDER	Basil, benzoin, bergamot, chamomile, clary sage, geranium, jasmine, lemon, lemon grass, mandarin, nutmeg, orange, patchouli, pine, rosemary, thyme		

NIAOULI	Coriander, fennel, juniper, lavender, lemon, lime, orange, pine, peppermint, rosemary	**ROSE**	Benzoin, bergamot, chamomile, clary sage, geranium, jasmine, lavender, neroli, orange, palmarosa, patchouli, sandalwood
NUTMEG	Other spices, cypress, frankincense, all citrus, patchouli, rosemary, tea tree	**ROSEMARY**	Basil, cedarwood, frankincense, geranium, ginger, grapefruit, lemon grass, lime, mandarin, melissa, orange, peppermint
ORANGE	Benzoin, cinnamon, coriander, clove, cypress, frankincense, geranium, jasmine, juniper, lavender, neroli, nutmeg, petitgrain, rose, rosewood	**ROSEWOOD**	Cedarwood, coriander, frankincense, geranium, palmarosa, patchouli, petitgrain, rose, rosemary, sandalwood, vetiver
PALMAROSA	Bergamot, citronella, geranium, jasmine, lavender, lime, melissa, orange, petitgrain, rose, rosewood, sandalwood, ylang-ylang	**SANDALWOOD**	Basil, benzoin, black pepper, cypress, frankincense, geranium, jasmine, lavender, lemon, myrrh, neroli, palmarosa, rose, vetiver, ylang-ylang
PATCHOULI	Bergamot, black pepper, clary sage, frankincense, geranium, ginger, lavender, lemon grass, myrrh, neroli, pine, rose, rosewood, sandalwood	**THYME**	Bergamot, cedarwood, chamomile, juniper, lemon, niaouli, mandarin, melissa, rosemary, tea tree
PEPPERMINT	Benzoin, cedarwood, cypress, lavender, mandarin, marjoram, niaouli, pine, rosemary	**TEA TREE**	Cinnamon, clove, cypress, eucalyptus, ginger, lavender, lemon, mandarin, orange, rosemary, thyme
PETITGRAIN	Benzoin, bergamot, cedarwood, geranium, lavender, melissa, neroli, orange, palmarosa, rosemary, rosewood, sandalwood, ylang-ylang	**VETIVER**	Benzoin, frankincense, geranium, grapefruit, jasmine, lavender, patchouli, rose, rosewood, sandalwood, ylang-ylang
PINE	Cedarwood, cinnamon, clove, cypress, eucalyptus, lavender, niaouli, rosemary, thyme, tea tree	**YLANG-YLANG**	Bergamot, grapefruit, jasmine, lavender, lemon, melissa, neroli, orange, patchouli, rose, rosewood, sandalwood, vetiver

THE PERFUMES OF ESSENTIAL OILS

It's useful to know in advance what a particular oil smells like in order to plan a balanced blend or to create a particular mood. Remember that the smell of the oil in the bottle is often quite different to the smell after exposure to air. The following comments are based on oil which has been on the skin for 30–40 seconds.

ANISEED *Pimpinella anisum*: Sweet and liquorice-like

BASIL *Ocimum basilicum*: Refreshing, uplifting and 'green'

BAY *Laurus nobilis*: Spicy

BENZOIN *Styrax benzoin*: Pleasant, warm, balsamic

BERGAMOT *Citrus bergamia*: Fresh, sweet and citrus-like

BLACK PEPPER *Piper nigrum*: Spicy, warm and 'woody'

CARAWAY *Carum carvi*: Warm, sweet and spicy

CARDAMOM *Elettaria cardamomum*: Sweet and spicy with a musky/woody undertone

CEDARWOOD *Juniperus virginiana*; *Cedrus atlantica*: Aromatic, warm

CHAMOMILE *Anthemis nobilis*; *Matricaria chamomilla* : Refreshing, pleasant and apple-like

CINNAMON *Cinnamomum zeylanicum*: Fragrant, spicy—similar to melissa

CITRONELLA *Cymbopogon nardus*: Clean and lemony

CLARY SAGE *Salvia sclarea*: Intoxicating, sweet, floral and fixative

CORIANDER *Coriandrum sativum*: Sweet, spicy with musky undertones

CLOVE *Eugenia carophyllus*: Pungent and spicy

CYPRESS *Cupressus sempervirens*: Clean and woody

EUCALYPTUS *Eucalyptus globulus* and other species: Clean, camphoraceous and cleansing

FENNEL *Foeniculum vulgare*: Similar to aniseed with floral overtones

FRANKINCENSE *Boswellia thurifera*; *B. Carterii*: Spicy and sweet

GERANIUM *Pelargonium odoratissima*; *P. graveolens*: Sweet, refreshing and relaxing; *P. graveolens* has a rose-like scent

GINGER *Zingiber officinalis*: Rich warm and spicy

GRAPEFRUIT *Citrus paradisi*: Fresh, sweet, sharp and altogether delightful!

HYSSOP *Hyssopus officinalis*: Spicy, warm, pungent and 'green'

JASMINE *Jasminum officinale, J. grandiflorum*: One of the most expensive. Exotic, sensual, relaxing

JUNIPER *Juniperus communis*: Sharp and stimulating

LAVENDER *Lavendula vera* and species: Fresh, clean, floral and soft

LEMON *Citrus limonum*: Sharp and fresh

LEMON GRASS *Cymbopogon citratus*: Strong earthy/citrus

LIME *Citrus aurantifolia*: Fresh, sweet and sharp

MANDARIN *Citrus reticulata*: Intense, sweet and tangy citrus scent

MARJORAM *Origanum marjorana*: Gently pungent and warm

MELISSA (LEMON BALM) *Melissa officinalis*: Clean, soft and lemony

MYRRH *Commiphora myrrha*: Smoky, musky, slightly acrid

NEROLI (ORANGE BLOSSOM) *Citrus vulgaris*: Sweet and ultra-feminine

NIAOULI *Melaleuca viridiflora*: Clear and camphoraceous

NUTMEG *Myristica fragrans*: Warm and spicy

ORANGE *Citrus vulgaris* and species: Happy, refreshing and sunny

PALMAROSA *Cymbopogon martinii*: Sweet with a rose-geranium like scent

PATCHOULI *Pogostemon patchouli*: Improves with age. Hot, heavy oriental perfume

PEPPERMINT *Mentha piperita*: Refreshing, penetrating minty scent

PETITGRAIN *Citrus bigardia*: Sweet with sharper undernotes of floral and citrus

PINE *Pinus sylvestris*: Resinous and clean

ROSE *Rosa centifolia; R. damascena; R. gallica*: Queen of perfumes—sensual and romantic

ROSEMARY *Rosmarinus officinalis*: Sharp and penetrating

ROSEWOOD *Aniba roseodora*: Floral and sweet with a woody undertone

SANDALWOOD *Santalum album*: Woody, spicy, oriental

TEA TREE *Melaleuca alternifolia*: Resinous, slightly musty

THYME *Thymus vulgaris*: Warmly, sweetly pungent

VETIVER *Vetiveria zizanioides*: Earthy, deep and persistent

YLANG-YLANG *Unona odorantissimum*: Sweet, sensual, exotic

COLOGNES, TOILET WATERS, AND PERFUMES

These preparations are some of the most exciting and possibly the most difficult ways of using essential oils.

Many of the great perfume houses use 100–200 different ingredients and take years to perfect a single perfume. Nevertheless you will find that you can make delicious perfumes which are tailored to you or your friends' personalities and which use only a few oils.

If you are serious about making perfumes you would be wise (as soon as you have your basic collection) to invest in a tiny amount of rose, jasmine and neroli oils. Even though these are very expensive it's possible to buy very small quantities and even one drop of these exquisite oils will make a profound difference to your finished product.

The most expensive perfumes usually contain extracts from the sex glands of animals, which create a sexual aura when incorporated in perfumes. These extracts are musk from the musk deer, ambergris from the sperm whale, civet from the civet cat, and castoreum from the beaver. I haven't included any of these objectionable additives in the following recipes.

The following tables should enable you to convert the blends to perfume, cologne and toilet water suitable for use as an 'after bath or shower splash'. I have deliberately not included any of the very expensive oils such as rose or jasmine as you probably won't be adding these to your stock until you have all the basic oils.

Colognes, toilet waters and perfumes all use essential oils, vodka or pure 70% proof alcohol, and purified water in varying amounts. Sometimes a little glycerine may be added to give body to splash toilet water and to counteract the drying effect of the alcohol.

Obviously the more essential oil used, the stronger the perfume.

The advantage of the less powerful colognes and toilet waters is that they may be used as a mist or splash over a larger area of the body, creating an 'aura' of light scent which is very appealing.

Do record everything you do as you create the masterpiece—the memory is notoriously fickle when it comes to remembering formulae.

The table headed 'Composition of Perfume, Cologne and Toilet Water' gives the amounts of oils, alcohol, water and glycerine to use. The quantities may be enlarged or reduced as you like but the proportions need to stay roughly the same.

COMPOSITION OF PERFUME, COLOGNE AND TOILET WATER

	ESSENTIAL OILS (ML)	ALCOHOL (ML)	WATER (ML)	GLYCERINE (ML)	TOTAL (ML)
PERFUME	5 ($\frac{1}{6}$fl oz)	10 ($\frac{1}{3}$fl oz)	0	0	15 ($\frac{1}{2}$fl oz)
COLOGNE	15 ($\frac{1}{2}$fl oz)	60 (2fl oz)	15 ($\frac{1}{2}$fl oz)	5 ($\frac{1}{6}$fl oz)	95 ($3\frac{1}{6}$fl oz)
TOILET WATER	10 ($\frac{1}{3}$fl oz)	100 ($3\frac{1}{3}$fl oz)	50 ($1\frac{2}{3}$fl oz)	10 ($\frac{1}{3}$fl oz)	170 ($5\frac{2}{3}$fl oz)

MAKING SCENTS

Now it's time to put some of the charts to use and blend some perfumes. Use tiny bottles when experimenting—I use a 10–15ml ($\frac{1}{3}$–$\frac{1}{2}$fl oz) dropper bottle. Begin with the base notes. Caution is the key as these will be the most long-lasting and dominant scents; in most perfumes the base note will need to be the least quantity unless you are seeking a heavy, sensual effect.

After the base notes add the middle notes, and finally the top notes to give the zing and freshness to the whole. Swirl the oils between each addition.

Then add the alcohol, swirl the contents, put the stopper in and leave for a couple of days before adding the water and glycerine.

Never test the smell directly from the bottle: put a drop on your wrist or a piece of blotting paper and wait a few moments before smelling. The smell at this stage will only give a rough approximation of the finished perfume as the mixture needs time to meld together and mature. Depending on the oils used and the complexity of the blend, this period can be anywhere from 6 weeks to 4 months or more.

The following recipes will help you to begin and to find out what appeals to you. They contain oils which are easy to obtain and aren't too expensive. Each recipe makes approximately 5ml (1 teaspoon) and lists the essential oils only.

The blend is now ready to use in any of the ways suggested in the recipes which follow or to make into perfume, cologne or toilet water using the table headed 'Composition of Perfume, Cologne and Toilet Water'.

Come Hither

40 drops ylang-ylang oil
15 drops patchouli oil
15 drops rose geranium oil
10 drops geranium oil
10 drops aniseed oil
10 drops bergamot oil

Combine the ylang-ylang and patchouli oils in a bottle. Add the rose geranium and geranium oils and swirl together. Finally add the aniseed and bergamot oils and mix well. Add the amount of alcohol needed for the type of product you want—see Composition of Perfumes, Colognes and Toilet Water in this chapter. Leave for 2 days, then add the water and glycerine needed.

Tassle from Linen and Lace of Balmain; flowers by Lisa Milasas

A selection of attractive perfume and cologne bottles

Misty New Moon

2 drops patchouli oil
4 drops clove oil
25 drops lavender oil
20 drops petitgrain oil
4 drops geranium oil
10 drops coriander oil
10 drops orange oil
10 drops lime oil
10 drops bergamot oil
10 drops vanilla essence

Combine the patchouli and clove oils in a bottle, add the lavender, petitgrain, geranium and coriander oils and swirl to mix. Finally, add the orange, lime and bergamot oils with the vanilla essence and mix well.

Add the amount of alcohol needed for the type of product you want—see Composition of Perfumes, Colognes and Toilet Water in this chapter. Leave for 2 days, then add the water and glycerine needed.

Satin Lady

4 drops patchouli oil
5 drops cinnamon oil
40 drops rose geranium oil
20 drops geranium oil
5 drops petitgrain oil
20 drops orange oil
5 drops lemon grass oil

Combine the patchouli and cinnamon oils in a bottle, add the rose geranium, geranium and petitgrain oils and swirl to mix. Finally, add the orange and lemon grass oils and mix well.

Add the amount of alcohol needed for the type of product you want—see Composition of Perfumes, Colognes and Toilet Water in this chapter. Leave for 2 days, then add the water and glycerine needed.

For Him Outdoors

30 drops cinnamon oil
2 drops frankincense oil
5 drops clove oil
5 drops petitgrain oil
30 drops bergamot oil
20 drops lime oil
10 drops vanilla essence

Combine the cinnamon, frankincense and clove oils in a bottle, add the petitgrain oil and swirl to mix. Finally, add the bergamot and lime oils with the vanilla essence and mix well.

Add the amount of alcohol needed for the type of product you want—see Composition of Perfumes, Colognes and Toilet Water in this chapter. Leave for 2 days, then add the water and glycerine needed.

Californian Dreaming

5 drops clove oil
5 drops sandalwood oil
5 drops petitgrain oil
10 drops rosemary oil
25 drops orange oil
30 drops lemon grass oil
20 drops lemon oil

Combine the clove and sandalwood oils in a bottle, add the petitgrain and rosemary oils and swirl to mix. Finally, add the orange, lemon grass and lemon oils and mix well.

Add the amount of alcohol needed for the type of product you want—see Composition of Perfumes, Colognes and Toilet Water in this chapter. Leave for 2 days, then add the water and glycerine needed.

Miss Victoria

10 drops cinnamon oil
8 drops petitgrain oil
2 drops rosemary oil
2 drops lavender oil
60 drops bergamot oil
10 drops lemon oil
10 drops vanilla essence

Combine the cinnamon, petitgrain, rosemary and lavender oils in a bottle and swirl to mix. Finally, add the bergamot and lemon oils with the vanilla essence and mix well.

Add the amount of alcohol needed for the type of product you want—see Composition of Perfumes, Colognes and Toilet Water in this chapter. Leave for 2 days, then add the water and glycerine needed.

Citrus Zinger

3 drops sandalwood oil
5 drops rosemary oil
5 drops petitgrain oil
45 drops orange oil
24 drops bergamot oil
20 drops lemon oil
3 drops peppermint oil

Combine the sandalwood, rosemary and petitgrain oils in a bottle and swirl to mix. Finally, add the orange, bergamot, lemon and peppermint oils and mix well.

Add the amount of alcohol needed for the type of product you want—see Composition of Perfumes, Colognes and Toilet Water in this chapter. Leave for 2 days, then add the water and glycerine needed.

Florida

4 drops cinnamon oil
4 drops clove oil
30 drops lavender oil
30 drops lemon oil
30 drops bergamot oil

Combine the cinnamon and clove oils in a bottle, add the lavender oil and swirl to mix. Finally, add the lemon and bergamot oils and mix well.

Add the amount of alcohol needed for the type of product you want—see Composition of Perfumes, Colognes and Toilet Water in this chapter. Leave for 2 days, then add the water and glycerine needed.

ESSENTIAL OILS FOR SKIN CARE

Essential oils are an ideal way to care for your skin and hair. They perform many functions, such as sebum regulation, cell regeneration and tissue firming. The following list will enable you to make substitutions in a recipe when you don't have a suggested oil or prefer the scent of another. Don't forget to consult the Classification of Essential Oils by Notes chart before making substitutions.

DRY SKIN

Benzoin, chamomile, carrot, evening primrose, frankincense, geranium, hyssop, jasmine, lavender, neroli, palmarosa, patchouli, rosemary, rose, sandalwood, ylang-ylang

NORMAL SKIN

Benzoin, chamomile, carrot, evening primrose, geranium, lemon, jasmine, neroli, lavender, palmarosa, patchouli, petitgrain, rose, rosemary, rosewood, sandalwood, ylang-ylang

OILY SKIN

Benzoin, bergamot, chamomile, carrot, clary sage, evening primrose, geranium, jasmine, lavender, lemon, lime, marjoram, melissa, neroli, petitgrain, rose, sandalwood, ylang-ylang

SENSITIVE SKIN

Chamomile, frankincense, jasmine, neroli, rose, sandalwood

MATURE SKIN

Cypress, frankincense, geranium, mandarin, palmarosa, rose, sandalwood, ylang-ylang

FOR PROBLEM SKIN

FOR PIMPLES
Benzoin, carrot, chamomile, clary sage, eucalyptus, evening primrose, geranium, juniper, lavender, lemon, patchouli, sandalwood,

FOR DEHYDRATED SKIN
Carrot, geranium, evening primrose, lavender, patchouli, sandalwood, peppermint

FOR ACNE
Carrot, chamomile, evening primrose, eucalyptus, geranium, lavender, tea tree, thyme

FOR ECZEMA
Carrot, chamomile, bergamot, eucalyptus, evening primrose, hyssop, lavender, patchouli

IRRITATED AND/OR INFLAMED SKIN
Chamomile, clary sage, jasmine, lavender, myrrh, patchouli, rose, tea tree

SCARS AND/OR STRETCH MARKS
Frankincense, lavender, mandarin, neroli, palmarosa, patchouli, rosewood, sandalwood

ESSENTIAL OILS FOR HAIR CARE

GENERAL HAIR CARE
Cedarwood, clary sage, geranium, lavender, rosemary
DRY HAIR
Chamomile, geranium, lavender, rosemary, sandalwood
OILY HAIR
Clary sage, cypress, eucalyptus, lavender, lemon, lime, rosemary, thyme
NORMAL HAIR
Lavender, lemon, geranium, rosemary
DANDRUFF
Cedarwood, clary sage, lavender, rosemary, sandalwood, thyme
FRAGILE HAIR
Chamomile, clary sage, lavender, sandalwood, thyme
LOSS OF HAIR
Cedarwood, juniper, lemon, melissa, palmarosa, rosemary
SCALP TONIC
Bay, cedarwood, chamomile, clary sage, lemon, nutmeg, rosemary, tea tree, ylang-ylang
SPLIT ENDS
Rosewood, sandalwood

OILS FOR STRESS-RELATED PROBLEMS

ANGER, ANXIETY   Basil, bergamot, chamomile, clary sage, cypress, frankincense, geranium, hyssop, jasmine, juniper, lavender, marjoram, melissa, neroli, ylang-ylang

DEPRESSION   Basil, clary sage, grapefruit, jasmine, lavender, melissa, neroli, rose, sandalwood, vetiver, ylang-ylang

INSOMNIA   Basil, chamomile, lavender, mandarin, marjoram, melissa, neroli, petitgrain, rose, sandalwood, thyme, ylang-ylang

NERVOUS EXHAUSTION   Basil, cinnamon, citronella, coriander, ginger, grapefruit, hyssop, jasmine, lavender, lemon grass, peppermint, nutmeg, rosemary, ylang-ylang

NERVOUS TENSION   Basil, bergamot, cedarwood, chamomile, cinnamon, frankincense, geranium, jasmine, lavender, marjoram, melissa, neroli, palmarosa, rosemary, vetiver, ylang-ylang

FRAGRANT OIL-BLENDS FOR HEALTH AND BEAUTY

Most recipes in this book contain essential oils but the following recipes are those in which the essential oils play a primary role of healing and beautifying instead of a secondary role of adding perfume.

Note: If you don't have the essential oil specified in the recipe, find substitutes in the preceding lists.

Example of suitable proportions for blends.
Base oils, to act as carrier.

86% almond oil, olive oil, grapeseed oil, herb oil (see Chapter One) or other fixed oil suitable for your skin type (see Chapter Two)

5% avocado oil—helps absorption of other oils and is highly nourishing

5% wheat germ oil—preservative, nutrient and emollient

2% evening primrose oil—nutrient and emollient

Add 2% essential oils, chosen from those suitable for your skin type

Total 100%

If you don't want to make 100ml ($3\frac{1}{3}$fl oz) you can use the above percentage example to make 50ml ($2\frac{2}{3}$fl oz) or less. Most of the following recipes are worked out on the above examples of 100ml ($3\frac{1}{3}$fl oz).

If you don't have oils such as evening primrose, jojoba or carrot it doesn't matter. It's perfectly all right to use more of the main oil, such as olive or almond, but do try to afford some wheat germ oil (not expensive) and include 5–10% to act as a preservative.

THE FACE

Essential oils mixed with rich, nourishing fruit, seed and nut oils make a perfect skin softening and moisturising treatment. As skin needs both oil and water the oils should be gently massaged into skin which has been lightly splashed or sprayed with water.

The essential oils in the recipes are only suggestions. By looking at the lists of Essential Oils for Skin Care, you will be able to personalise your own luxurious skin treatment.

Regenerating Oil for Dry Skin

$\frac{1}{3}$ cup (80ml/$2\frac{2}{3}$fl oz) almond oil
1 teaspoon olive oil
40 drops carrot oil
40 drops jojoba oil
1 teaspoon wheat germ oil
15 drops palmarosa oil
5 drops lavender oil
5 drops sandalwood oil
5 drops ylang-ylang oil

Combine all the ingredients in a 100ml ($3\frac{1}{3}$fl oz) bottle. Shake well for several minutes. Leave for 4 days to blend. Store in a cool dark place. Shake before use. Gently massage into your skin, which has been lightly sprayed with water, each morning and night.

Regenerating Oil for Oily Skin

Those of you with oily skin will have noticed that there are areas on your face and neck which have little or no oil: these are mainly the throat, lips and under the eyes. Use the oil on these areas but also use a thin smear over the whole face before going to bed as the essential oils have the capacity for 'balancing' and moisturising the skin without encouraging the oil glands to produce more sebum.

⅓ cup (80ml/2⅔fl oz) grapeseed oil
2 teaspoons apricot oil
40 drops evening primrose oil
40 drops carrot oil
10 drops bergamot oil
5 drops lemon oil
5 drops lavender oil
10 drops sandalwood

Combine all the ingredients in a 100ml (3⅓fl oz) bottle. Shake well for several minutes. Leave for 4 days to blend. Store in a cool dark place. Shake before use.

Regenerating Oil for Normal Skin

Rarely found after the blessed state of babyhood has been left behind—but those of you fortunate enough to possess firm, smooth, fine-textured skin with no 'broken' veins should make a big effort to keep it this way. This oil will help.

⅓ cup (80ml/2⅔fl oz) almond oil
1 teaspoon avocado oil
1 teaspoon wheat germ oil
1 teaspoon jojoba oil
5 drops lavender oil
15 drops palmarosa oil
5 drops rosewood oil
5 drops sandalwood oil

Combine all the ingredients in a 100ml (3⅓fl oz) bottle. Shake well for several minutes. Leave for 4 days to blend. Store in a cool dark place. Shake before use.

Regenerating Oil for Sensitive Skin

This blend contains only 0.5% of the gentlest essential oils. Nevertheless, test all the oils on another part of your skin before blending and using on your face. Refer to the instructions for patch testing under 'Allergen' in the Glossary.

⅓ cup (80ml/2⅔fl oz) almond oil
3 teaspoons apricot oil
40 drops evening primrose oil
20 drops chamomile oil
5 drops frankincense oil
5 drops geranium oil

Combine all the ingredients in a 100ml (3⅓fl oz) bottle. Shake well for several minutes. Leave for 4 days to blend. Store in a cool dark place. Shake before use.

ACNE

Problems such as acne and blackheads are dealt with in depth in Chapter Two but the following oils and lotions are also very important in the treatment of these conditions.

Herbal Rinse Lotion

90ml (3fl oz) cider vinegar
15 drops lavender oil
15 drops tea tree oil
2 teaspoons tincture of myrrh

Combine all the ingredients in a 100ml (3⅓fl oz) bottle. Shake well for several minutes. Leave for 4 days to blend. Store in a cool dark place. Shake before use.

Shake the mixture. Add 1 teaspoon to 1 cup (250ml/8fl oz) warm water and use as a final rinse after washing the face.

Herbal Healing Day Oil

This gentle but powerful oil is for day treatment of acne, pimples or otherwise infected skin.

40ml (1⅓fl oz) almond oil
20 drops carrot oil
5 drops tea tree oil
5 drops lavender oil
2 drops thyme oil
5 drops geranium oil

Combine all the ingredients in a 50ml (2⅔fl oz) bottle. Shake well for several minutes. Leave for 4 days to blend. Store in a cool dark place.

Shake mixture. Put 3–4 drops on the palm of your hand, dip the fingers in and gently smooth over the skin. Don't get any in the eyes or it will sting. Leave on for 5–10 minutes, blot surplus off with tissue. Use morning and midday.

Herbal Healing Night Oil

This blend feels a little oilier than its daytime sister but don't worry—these oils work while you sleep, to soothe, heal and regenerate, as a night treatment for acne and pimples.

40ml (1⅓fl oz) almond oil
20 drops carrot oil
20 drops evening primrose oil
5 drops tea tree oil
5 drops chamomile or lavender oil

Combine all the ingredients in a 50ml (2⅔fl oz) bottle. Shake well for several minutes. Leave for 4 days to blend. Store in a cool dark place.

Apply the same amount and in the same way as the Herbal Healing Day Oil.

Cleansing Facial Steam

The antibacterial action of this treatment combined with the heat from the steam will draw impurities to the surface so don't do it before a big date!

1 teaspoon bergamot oil
1 teaspoon lavender oil
½ teaspoon tea tree oil
20 drops thyme oil
30 drops geranium oil

Combine all the ingredients in a 15ml (½fl oz) bottle. Shake well for several minutes. Leave for 4 days to blend. Store in a cool dark place.

Add 10 drops of the blended oils to a bowl of boiling water. Hold your face 35cm (14in) above the water and cover your head with a towel forming a tent over the bowl. Stay in your tent for a maximum of 5 minutes.

THE NECK

The skin on the neck seems to age faster than anywhere else on the body. It's difficult to spend all your life wearing a scarf to hide the crinkles and wrinkles so we should spend at least as much—if not more—time and effort caring for this often neglected but very exposed part of ourselves. Cleansing, toning and moisturising the neck will ensure that we are doing the best we can to keep the skin in as good a condition as our faces.

Oil for the Neck

This oil blend is very powerful and should be used at night to get the best result.

2 teaspoons avocado oil

2 teaspoons evening primrose oil

2 tablespoons wheat germ oil

1 tablespoon almond oil

1 teaspoon jojoba oil

20 drops carrot oil

15 drops palmarosa oil

5 drops rosewood oil

5 drops frankincense oil

5 drops geranium oil

Combine all the ingredients in a 100ml (3$\frac{1}{3}$fl oz) bottle. Shake well for several minutes. Leave for 4 days to blend. Store in a cool dark place.

Shake mixture. Measure 5–10 drops into the palm of your hand and, using a light, upward motion, use the fingers of the other hand to spread the oil from the collarbones to the chin. Massage in, leave 20 minutes and blot the surplus off with a tissue.

AROUND THE EYES

The thin, fine skin around the eyes shows early lines in the same way as the neck. Crow's-feet, bags under the eyes and dark circles can be very demoralising—laughter and smile lines are a different matter!

A famous actress when being photographed is said to have refused to allow the use of filters on the camera to disguise her facial lines. She said that she had lived very enthusiastically and hard to earn the lines and was proud of them all!

Remember that the skin around the eyes is super fragile and more harm than good can be done if you are heavy-handed. Use only the middle finger to gently pat oils, creams and lotions on this area and avoid using heavy oils which can 'drag'.

Around-the-eyes Oil

This is an oil suitable for all age groups.

45ml (1$\frac{1}{2}$fl oz) almond oil

15 drops jojoba oil

35 drops evening primrose oil

15 drops carrot oil

5 drops lemon oil

5 drops lavender oil

3 x 250 IU capsules vitamin E oil

Combine all the ingredients in a 50ml (2$\frac{2}{3}$fl oz) bottle. Prick the vitamin E capsules and squeeze into the bottle. Shake the bottle really well to mix. Leave for 4 days to blend. Store in a cool dark place.

Shake the mixture well. One drop for under each eye should be enough. Apply the oil at night, leave for 10 minutes and carefully blot the excess off with a tissue. Avoid getting the oil into the eye itself or it will sting and could be harmful.

HANDS AND NAILS

Use the following oil every day if possible. Our hands and nails are often subjected to more abuse than any other part of our bodies and are often given less attention. Treat yourself to a home manicure once a week and make an effort to use rubber gloves as often as you can, particularly for washing up as detergent takes all the oil out of skin and makes nails brittle.

'Shalimar' Hand and Nail Oil

1 tablespoon almond oil
1 tablespoon apricot oil
30 drops evening primrose oil
30 drops carrot oil
30 drops jojoba oil
15 drops palmarosa oil
5 drops rosewood oil
5 drops geranium oil
2 drops sandalwood oil
4 x 250 IU capsules vitamin E oil

Combine all the ingredients in a 50ml ($2^{2}/_{3}$fl oz) bottle (prick the vitamin E capsules and squeeze into the bottle). Shake the bottle really well to mix. Leave for 4 days to blend. Store in a cool dark place.

Shake the bottle well before use. Massage 4–5 drops in well; repeat if liked.

FEET

Herbal Foot Oil

Your feet will thank you for massaging them with this beautiful oil. Not only does it ease the pain of tired feet but it also helps to cure tinea and other diseases of the skin on the feet.

1 tablespoon vodka
40ml ($1^{1}/_{3}$fl oz) olive oil
2 teaspoons avocado oil
2 teaspoons wheat germ oil
2 teaspoons almond oil
20 drops lavender oil
10 drops cypress oil
5 drops rosemary oil
5 drops tea tree oil

Combine all the ingredients in a 100ml ($3^{1}/_{3}$fl oz) bottle. Shake well for several minutes. Leave for 4 days to blend. Store in a cool dark place.

Wash or soak the feet first, then dry thoroughly. Shake the bottle well and massage a little of the oil into the feet until absorbed.

HAIR

Hair dressings keep the hair glossy and smooth.

Herbal Hair Dressing 1
FOR ALL HAIR TYPES

2 teaspoons rosemary oil
2 teaspoons lavender oil
50 drops basil oil
50 drops thyme oil

Combine all ingredients in a 25ml (about 1fl oz) bottle. Shake well. Leave for 4 days to blend. Store in a cool dark place.

Shake the mixture well. Put a few drops on the palm of your hand and rub the hands together. Now rub the oil from your palms through your hair. This can be done as often as you like.

Herbal Hair Dressing 2

FOR DRY HAIR

If you don't have basil oil, the lavender oil may be increased to 2 teaspoons.

2 teaspoons rosemary oil
1 teaspoon jojoba oil
1 teaspoon lavender oil
1 teaspoon basil oil

Combine all ingredients in a 25ml (about 1fl oz) bottle. Shake well. Leave for 4 days to blend. Store in a cool dark place.

Shake the mixture well. Put a few drops on the palm of your hand and rub the hands together. Now rub the oil from your palms thoroughly through your hair.

BATHS

There are many different types of baths in which we may use essential oils beneficially—foot, hand, sitz, half, full.

The preparations below are enough for one bath. When you find a blend you really enjoy you can mix larger quantities as oil blends improve with age.

Antibacterial and Antiviral

3 drops tea tree oil
3 drops eucalyptus oil
3 drops lavender oil
1 drop thyme oil

Mix the ingredients with either 1 tablespoon full cream milk or vegetable oil. Add the mixture to the bath after the bath has been run. 'Swoosh' well to disperse.

Deodorant Bath Oil

4 drops clary sage oil
2 drops bergamot oil
2 drops patchouli oil
2 drops geranium oil

Mix the ingredients with either 1 tablespoon full cream milk or vegetable oil. Add the mixture to the bath after the bath has been run. 'Swoosh' well to disperse.

Moisturising Oil for Dry Skin

4 drops chamomile oil
4 drops geranium oil
2 drops palmarosa oil

Mix the ingredients with either 1 tablespoon full cream milk or vegetable oil. Add the mixture to the bath after the bath has been run. 'Swoosh' well to disperse.

Oily Skin Control

5 drops lemon oil
3 drops bergamot oil
2 drops rosewood oil

Mix the ingredients with either 1 tablespoon full cream milk or vegetable oil. Add the mixture to the bath after the bath has been run. 'Swoosh' well to disperse.

Dew Drops Hydrating Bath Oil

2 drops chamomile oil
2 drops lavender oil
2 drops carrot oil
2 drops geranium oil
2 drops palmarosa oil (optional)

Mix the ingredients with either 1 tablespoon full cream milk or vegetable oil. Add the mixture to the bath after the bath has been run. 'Swoosh' well to disperse.

Feeling Fantastic

4 drops grapefruit oil

2 drops geranium oil

2 drops ylang-ylang oil

2 drops patchouli oil

Mix the ingredients with either 1 tablespoon full cream milk or vegetable oil. Add to the bath after the bath has been run. 'Swoosh' well to disperse.

Pick-me-up

4 drops lavender oil

3 drops rosemary oil

2 drops black pepper oil

Mix the ingredients with either 1 tablespoon full cream milk or vegetable oil. Add the mixture to the bath after the bath has been run. 'Swoosh' well to disperse.

Relaxing

4 drops marjoram oil

3 drops lavender oil

3 drops ylang-ylang oil

Mix the ingredients with either 1 tablespoon full cream milk or vegetable oil. Add the mixture to the bath after the bath has been run. 'Swoosh' well to disperse.

Break of Day

3 drops grapefruit oil

3 drops lemon oil

2 drops bergamot oil

2 drops peppermint oil

Mix the ingredients with either 1 tablespoon full cream milk or vegetable oil. Add the mixture to the bath after the bath has been run. 'Swoosh' well to disperse.

Sweet Dreams

4 drops chamomile oil

2 drops lavender oil

2 drops marjoram oil

2 drops sandalwood oil

Mix the ingredients with either 1 tablespoon full cream milk or vegetable oil. Add the mixture to the bath after the bath has been run. 'Swoosh' well to disperse.

MASSAGE OILS

Basic Massage Oil

To make 100ml ($3\frac{1}{3}$fl oz) massage oil the following formula can be used but the types of oils (apart from the Herb Oil Base) may be changed depending on individual need and availability. I always use a triple strength herb oil base as the main oil in a massage oil blend.

70ml ($2\frac{1}{3}$fl oz) Herb Oil Base

(see Chapter One)

2 teaspoons almond oil

2 teaspoons avocado oil

1 teaspoon wheat germ oil

Combine all the ingredients in a 100ml ($3\frac{1}{3}$fl oz) bottle. Shake well to mix.

The following recipes are suggestions for suitable blends of pure essential oils to add to the Basic Massage Oil.

The blends listed in the Baths section in this chapter, may also be used for massage oils. Use 40–60 drops of these blends to each 100ml ($3\frac{1}{3}$fl oz) of Basic Massage Oil.

Stressed-out Bodies

A good blend for those times when you ache all over.

20 drops lavender oil
10 drops rosemary oil
10 drops black pepper oil
5 drops peppermint oil
5 drops cypress oil

Add the ingredients to the entire bottle of Basic Massage Oil. Shake well to mix.

Stressed-out Minds

When you are mentally exhausted and sick of thinking this blend will allow you to fade far away, relax and forget for a while.

10 drops bergamot oil
20 drops geranium oil
10 drops ylang-ylang oil
5 drops frankincense oil
5 drops cedarwood oil

Add the ingredients to the entire bottle of Basic Massage Oil. Shake well to mix.

For Lovers

10 drops petitgrain or neroli oil
20 drops ylang-ylang oil
10 drops rose geranium or rose oil
10 drops patchouli oil

Add the ingredients to the entire bottle of Basic Massage Oil. Shake well to mix.

Rondoletia

The blend to pamper and soothe you after a hard day.

20 drops lavender oil
20 drops rose geranium or rose oil
10 drops clove oil

Add the ingredients to the entire bottle of Basic Massage Oil. Shake well to mix.

Night's Ease

To relieve stress and ensure a restful relaxed night's sleep.

10 drops chamomile oil
10 drops ylang-ylang oil
10 drops marjoram oil
10 drops sandalwood oil

Add the ingredients to the entire bottle of Basic Massage Oil. Shake well to mix.

To Ease Rheumatism and Arthritis

Massage is a useful part of an all-over treatment for painful complaints of rheumatoid arthritis and osteoarthritis.

20 drops cedarwood oil
15 drops lavender oil
10 drops black pepper oil
5 drops rosemary oil

Add the ingredients to the entire bottle of Basic Massage Oil. Shake well to mix.

PERFUMES FOR THE HOME

When they make compound perfumes, they moisten the spices with fragrant wine.
—Theophrastus (c. 4th century–c. 3rd century BC)

ROOM SPRAYS

There are many reasons for using oils in room sprays, including to perfume and freshen; and as bacterial/viral/insect repellents, ionisers and energy-raisers.

Air-freshener blends may be used in diffusers, or a few drops may be placed on light globes, radiators and other warm places.

The air in a heated room can get very dry, which in turn can dry the skin. Humidify and freshen the air by putting a few drops of essential-oil blend in a small bowl of water and placing the bowl near the heat source.

In the following recipes you will need a spray bottle of at least 300ml (10fl oz) capacity, 50ml (1⅔fl oz) alcohol and 1 cup (250ml/8fl oz) purified water. You will only be using a little of the oil blends at a time, so the remainder should be stored in a cool dark place.

Sitting-room Freshener

This blend will act as a relaxing air freshener but will also help to keep at bay viruses and bacteria brought in by visitors.

2 teaspoons lavender oil
1 teaspoon rose geranium oil
1 teaspoon bergamot oil
40 drops cinnamon oil
40 drops sandalwood oil

Mix all the oils in a 25ml (about 1fl oz) bottle. Store in a cool dark place.

Shake the bottle. Take 1 teaspoon (5ml) of this oil blend and add to 50ml (1⅔fl oz) alcohol in a spray bottle of at least 300ml (10fl oz) capacity. Allow the oil to dissolve, then add 1 cup (250ml/8fl oz) purified water. Shake bottle well before using.

Bedroom Blend

To create a relaxed, restful aura in the bedroom.

40 drops chamomile oil
1 teaspoon geranium oil
2 teaspoons bergamot oil
40 drops frankincense oil
40 drops ylang-ylang oil
40 drops patchouli oil

Mix all the oils in a 25ml (about 1fl oz) bottle. Store in a cool dark place.

Shake the bottle. Take 1 teaspoon (5ml) of this oil blend and add to 50ml (1⅔fl oz) alcohol in a spray bottle of at least 300ml (10fl oz) capacity. Allow the oil to dissolve, then add 1 cup (250ml/8fl oz) purified water. Shake well before using. Use sparingly.

Anti-Mosquito Blend

This blend may be used both on the body and in the air to keep mosquitoes at bay. See also Blending and Diluting the Oils information earlier in this chapter.

> 2 teaspoons citronella oil
> 1 teaspoon lemon grass oil
> 1 teaspoon lavender oil
> 1 teaspoon cedarwood oil

Mix all the oils in a 25ml (about 1fl oz) bottle. Store in a cool dark place.

TO USE IN AN AIR SPRAY: Shake the bottle. Take 1 teaspoon (5ml) of this oil blend and add to 50ml (1²⁄₃fl oz) alcohol in a spray bottle of at least 300ml (10fl oz) capacity. Allow the oil to dissolve, then add 1 cup (250ml/8fl oz) purified water. Shake well before using.

TO USE ON THE BODY: Put 25 drops in a 50ml (1²⁄₃fl oz) bottle, add 2 teaspoons vodka or witch hazel, and fill with grapeseed or almond oil. Shake well before rubbing onto exposed parts of the body.

OTHER USES

Some people believe the oil blends listed below have magical properties, and some use the blends to facilitate 'visualisation' (i.e. the calling up of mental images).

These oil blends may be used in diffusers, incense and sprays, or for sniffing (use a few drops on cotton wool)—they are not for drinking. Oils diffuse nicely into the air if a few drops are placed on cold light globes (then turn on), warm radiators, wood in open fires and anywhere that there is heat.

Don't worry if you don't have all the oils in a recipe. It's perfectly all right to increase the amounts of the other oils or to choose oils with similar qualities.

The following blends should be mixed in a 25ml (1fl oz) bottle, store in a cool dark place.

To raise consciousness: 1 teaspoon basil oil, 1 teaspoon hyssop oil, 1 teaspoon lavender oil, 40 drops pennyroyal oil, 40 drops sage oil, 1 teaspoon thyme oil.

To instil courage: 2 teaspoons clove oil, 2 teaspoons fennel oil, 1 teaspoon thyme oil.

To lift depression: 1 teaspoon basil oil, 1 teaspoon clary sage oil, 1 teaspoon melissa oil, 2 teaspoons ylang-ylang oil.

To create protection: 2 teaspoons basil oil, 40 drops clove oil, 2 teaspoons petitgrain oil, 40 drops geranium oil.

To induce psychic power: 2 teaspoons bay oil, 1 teaspoon lemon grass oil, 40 drops cinnamon oil, 40 drops yarrow oil, 1 teaspoon nutmeg oil.

To purify: 1 teaspoon hyssop oil, 1 teaspoon juniper oil, 1 teaspoon camphor oil, 40 drops lemon grass oil, 40 drops orange oil.

To heal: 1 teaspoon eucalyptus oil, 1 teaspoon tea tree oil, 1 teaspoon cypress oil, 1 teaspoon pine oil, 1 teaspoon sandalwood oil.

To bring love: 1 teaspoon rosemary oil, 1 teaspoon lavender oil, 40 drops coriander oil, 40 drops lemon verbena oil, 2 teaspoons ylang-ylang oil.

To raise magical powers: 1 teaspoon nutmeg oil, 1 teaspoon bay oil, 1 teaspoon orange oil, 1 teaspoon sage oil.

To bring money: 2 teaspoons basil oil, 2 teaspoons sage oil, 40 drops patchouli oil, 40 drops nutmeg oil.

To arouse sexual desire: 1 teaspoon sandalwood oil, 2 teaspoons ylang-ylang oil, 1 teaspoon lavender oil, 40 drops patchouli oil, 40 drops rosemary oil, 10 drops rose oil.

For spirituality: 1 teaspoon cedar oil, 2 teaspoons sandalwood oil, 1 teaspoon myrrh oil, 1 teaspoon frankincense oil.

For the brain and memory: 2 teaspoons rosemary oil, 2 teaspoons sage oil, 1 teaspoon clove oil.

CHAPTER SEVEN

FOOD AND THE BALANCED DIET

These days we are faced with a dichotomy. Health authorities are

urging us to eat less fat and more grains, fruit and vegetables but

'fast food' outlets continue to flourish and convenience foods

flood the supermarket shelves. More than ever before, the

caregiver in the family (whether man or woman) works outside

the home for financial or other reasons. This can create

enormous physical, emotional and mental stress. The time and

energy available to spend on shopping and cooking is minimal but

at the same time we want to do the best we can for our families.

*Many of the necessary foods
to create a balanced diet*

EATING WELL

I have been a 'mother and money earner' for most of my adult life and am very aware of the appeal of 'takeaway' and convenience foods; when you are exhausted at the end of a hard day, these foods are a real temptation and are not going to do much harm if indulged in very occasionally.

The main criticism of fast food is that it contains too much fat, sugar and salt and too little fibre, vitamins and minerals. It's obvious that the safest, cheapest, tastiest and healthiest foods are those which you prepare and cook yourself from unprocessed ingredients.

In order to be healthy we need to eat foods, in the correct proportions, from all the food groups: carbohydrates (including fibre), protein, and fats. We also need vitamins, minerals and trace elements, and water.

CARBOHYDRATES

What are carbohydrates and what do they do?

Carbohydrates are fuel which provides energy and 'staying power' for your body. Until the last few years, carbohydrates were seen as 'fattening'. Certainly, if eaten in quantities larger than the body needs, they are stored as fat, but so are excesses of protein and fats. Dietary fibres are also carbohydrate and form what is known as 'roughage'.

Carbohydrates are divided into three main groups: complex carbohydrates, sugars, and fibre.

COMPLEX CARBOHYDRATES

This group includes bread, vegetables, cereals, fruit and legumes. Complex carbohydrates are digested to become glucose which if not utilised immediately as energy is stored as glycogen in the liver to be used as an energy reserve. Any excess is stored as fat. It is more desirable to obtain energy from complex carbohydrates.

SUGARS

During digestion, sugars are broken down and absorbed into the bloodstream as glucose—the primary fuel for the brain. The various sugars are:

(a) sucrose obtained mainly from sugar cane;
(b) glucose found in sweet fruits, honey and corn;
(c) fructose present in ripe fruits, honey and some vegetables;
(d) maltose found in grains such as barley and wheat; and
(e) lactose found only in milk.

REFINED SUGAR

Sugar is included in a large proportion of the foods we eat. We use sugar in cooking cakes, biscuits, and in sauces. We add it to tea, coffee and cordials. Soft drinks and many alcoholic drinks have a high sugar content.

Look for 'hidden' sugar when you go shopping. If you begin to read labels you will be surprised to find how many items contain sugar.

Labels can mislead people (those who are unfamiliar with the different types of sugar) into believing that a product is sugar-free by using the following names: lactose, glucose, maltose, levulose, invertase, corn syrup, maple syrup, dextrose, fructose and sucrose. When you see any of these you will know that sugar has been added!

People often depend on refined sugar or sweets containing refined sugar to replace lost energy. The 'minus' side of this is that it can lower your blood sugar to less than its previous level, leaving you more tired, hungry and depressed than you were originally.

Fruits, vegetables, cereals and grains contain starches and sugars which are converted more slowly into glucose and glycogen. As the release is slower, energy lasts for a long time without giving the 'low' associated with refined sugar intake.

Excessive refined sugar intake has been associated with increased tooth plaque and tooth decay, anaemia, kidney lesions, dermatitis, weight gain, high blood pressure and heart problems.

FIBRE

There is much talk about fibre (or lack of it) in the Western diet. Dietary fibre is a carbohydrate made up of the material which forms the cell-wall of plants. Insoluble fibre such as wheat bran can't be digested by body enzymes and passes as roughage through our bodies. Soluble fibre present in oats, legumes, fruits etc is digested by bacteria—producing valuable acids in the process.

WHAT DOES FIBRE DO?

Insoluble fibre does most of its work in the bowel where it holds water and shortens the length of time taken by food to leave the body. This means that stools are soft and bulky—easier to release.

If the diet is lacking in fibre the stools become hard and dry, and constipation will result. Soluble fibre such as oat bran helps to control blood sugar and cholesterol levels.

Research has shown that lack of fibre in our foods may lead to obesity, piles, diverticulitis (small pouches which form in the wall of the bowel caused, in part, by the effort of excreting hard faeces) and bowel cancer.

WHERE DO WE FIND FIBRE?

It's not good enough to sprinkle large amounts of raw wheat bran over your breakfast cereal. Indeed it could be harmful—more than 2 tablespoons a day could irritate the gut and cause nutrient imbalance The elderly or those with coeliac disease may not tolerate any wheat bran at all.

FIBRE CONTENT OF SOME FOODS

FOOD	SERVING SIZE	GRAMS OF FIBRE
Almond kernels	28g (1oz)	4.1
Apple, raw	1 average	2.1
Baked beans in tomato sauce	224g (7oz) can	16.5
Banana	1 average	3.4
Bran	2 tablespoons	6.0
Broccoli head, steamed	112g (3½oz)	4.6
Brown rice, uncooked	56g (2oz)	2.4
Carrots	112g (3½oz)	3.4
Dried fruit	50g (1⅔oz)	9.0
Fresh or frozen peas	112g (3½oz)	9.1
Jacket potato, with skin	224g (7oz)	5.0
Lentils, uncooked	42g (1½oz)	5.0
Muesli	56g (2oz)	4.2
Orange	1 average	2.5
Peanut butter	30g (1oz)	3.0
Red kidney beans, cooked	200g (6½oz)	18.0
Spinach	112g (3½oz)	7.1
Sweetcorn kernels	112g (3½oz)	5.7
White rice	56g (2oz)	1.4
Wholemeal bread	2 thin slices	5.0

PROTEIN

Our skin, hair, nails, tendons, muscles and cartilages form the 20% protein of which our bodies are composed. Proteins are needed for the building and replacement of body cells and for the production of some hormones and enzymes. Proteins are composed of amino acids—about twenty-two different ones.

There are eight essential amino acids which cannot be synthesised by the body and must be obtained from outside sources. Not all protein foods contain the eight essential amino acids.

WHERE DO WE FIND PROTEIN?

'Complete' proteins (with all essential amino acids) are obtained from fish, meat, cheese, milk, eggs, tofu (soya bean curd) and tempeh (fermented soya beans).

Most grains and pulses (with the exception of soya beans and some sprouted grains) are incomplete proteins but may be made complete by mixing them—such as bread and hummus.

Some authorities feel that it's desirable to obtain some of our daily protein requirements from fish, meat or eggs and the remainder from legumes; however, from my observation, if a vegetarian diet is well and carefully planned with special attention being paid to an adequate intake of iron and vitamin B$_{12}$, it is very healthy.

HOW MUCH DO WE NEED?

An excess of protein is stored as fat which can result in heart disease, obesity and other conditions. The daily allowance for an 'average' person could be as little as 300ml (10fl oz) skim milk, 60g (2oz) lean meat, 60g (2oz) wholegrain cereals, 30g (1oz) cottage cheese and 1 egg.

Children, adolescents, pregnant and lactating women, the elderly and vegetarians need more protein. If you are mentally or physically stressed, play lots of sport, or work in a hot climate where you perspire a lot, you may need more protein.

OILS AND FATS

Oil and fats come from sources which include:

(a) The visible oils and fats we use such as butter, margarine, vegetables, nut, fruit and seed oils and animals fats; and

(b) The invisible oils and fats found in fish, meat, eggs, cheese, cream, grains and some fruit and vegetables.

Our bodies do need some fat (notably, polyunsaturated and monounsaturated fatty acids) in the diet in order to develop many body processes. Other fats are made by the body from carbohydrates and proteins.

It seems that the people who regularly eat too much fat also eat too little fibre—a recipe for obesity, heart attacks, constipation and ill health.

Carbohydrates and proteins contain 16.8 kilojoules (70 calories) per gram. Fat contains 37.8 kilojoules (158 calories) per gram so, if you have a weight problem, by cutting down on fats you will automatically lose weight.

It is recommended that only 30% of our total daily kilojoules (calories) should be derived from fat (less for those people who have cholesterol or weight problems). Other authorities feel that 20% is safer; 15% would result in a reduction in blood cholesterol levels and obesity if combined with a suitably high fibre diet.

The easiest way for people who have normal weight/height ratio (meaning that they're neither too fat nor too thin) to watch their daily fat intake is as follows:

➤ Restrict meat portions to 75–125g (2½–4oz) daily (mainly chicken and fish, beef only occasionally—all visible fat and skin removed).
➤ Use only 1 tablespoon butter daily.
➤ Drink skim milk.
➤ Eat low-fat cheeses and yoghurt.
➤ Cut the oils used in cooking to a minimum. If a recipe says 2 tablespoons oil, try 2 teaspoons. Use monounsaturated oils—olive and canola.
➤ Eat no more than 3 whole eggs a week. Use only the egg whites for coating fish, patties etc.

Use cold-pressed oils and good quality vinegars

VITAMINS AND MINERALS

Vitamins and minerals are natural substances present in minute amounts in food. They are not substitutes for proteins, carbohydrates and fats; in fact, vitamins and minerals need these nutrients (and vice versa!) in order to be assimilated into the body. They don't provide energy but are essential for the energy from food to be made available to the body.

Vitamins are also responsible for the assimilation of some minerals. Minerals, in their turn, are a necessary aid to the assimilation and functioning of vitamins. They also provide the body with necessary elements. Without a balanced diet, the most assiduous taking of supplements will not give you good health.

You will probably need extra vitamins and/or minerals if you are: under stress; working in an unhealthy environment; a drinker or smoker; recovering from an illness/operation; or on a reducing diet of less than 5000 kilojoules (1200 calories). You can either increase your intake of the appropriate foods or see a nutritionist who will be able to suggest supplements.

In the following pages I give suggestions for foods richest in particular vitamins and minerals. If you never or rarely eat these foods, your intake of vitamins and minerals may be lacking. The best way to remedy this deficiency is to begin adding these foods daily.

Some vitamins—notably vitamin C—are very fragile and may be partially or totally lost due to canning, bottling, freezing, overlong storage, soaking or overcooking and reheating of fruit and vegetables.

Picking your own garden-fresh vegetables and lightly steaming them or eating many of them raw, as well as eating at least two pieces of fruit a day, should ensure that daily vitamin C requirements are met.

Minerals can leach out into cooking water so it's very important to use the water for soups and stock, or with tomato juice, as a drink.

I don't suggest any recommended daily intake as the amounts required are very debatable (and also very small). Every country seems to have a different recommended dietary intake (RDI) table; every human being is unique and each person's RDI will vary according to his or her own nutritional requirements.

VITAMINS

Vitamins fall into two categories: those which are water-soluble, and those which are fat-soluble.

WATER-SOLUBLE

These are vitamin C and the eight B complex vitamins. 'Water-soluble' means that these vitamins can be lost to the water during cooking and can be passed in urine if present in excess to the needs of the body. The body doesn't store these and ideally they should be replaced daily.

FAT-SOLUBLE

Vitamins A, D, E and K are soluble both in food fats and body fat. They are stored in the body, making it possible to create a 'build-up' with attendant problems. A regular supply of fat-soluble vitamins is less crucial.

When you make your food choices, note the difference between 'water-soluble' vitamins which need replacing every day and 'fat-soluble' vitamins which are stored in the body. Take note also of the number of vitamins which are wholly or partially destroyed by processing.

VITAMIN A
FAT-SOLUBLE

Excessive intake may be harmful.

SOME BENEFITS Counteracts night blindness. Improves poor eyesight. Needed for growth and reproduction. Aids recovery from illness.

Keeps the mucous tissue lining the mouth, respiratory and urinary tracts in normal condition. Protects against some cancers.

MAIN FOOD SOURCES Liver; fish oils; eggs; milk; butter; orange and dark green vegetables.

HERB SOURCES Very high: alfalfa, dandelion greens, nettle (young leaves), watercress. Other: calendula, elecampane, lettuce, spearmint, parsley, violet leaves, yellow dock root.

THE B VITAMINS

The eight best known B vitamins work in conjunction with each other and shouldn't be taken as isolated vitamins without ensuring that your diet is rich in the remaining ones.

VITAMIN B$_1$ (THIAMIN)
WATER-SOLUBLE

Alcoholics may need extra.

SOME BENEFITS Helps digestion of carbohydrates. Helps to improve mental outlook. May combat air- and sea-sickness. Useful to diabetics, elderly people, alcoholics and those who eat a lot of 'junk' food.

MAIN FOOD SOURCES Wholegrains, bran, organ meats, beef, molasses, nuts, tofu, brewer's yeast, soya beans, sunflower seeds, wheat germ, skim milk, eggs, sprouted seeds and grains.

HERB SOURCES Very high: dandelion greens, watercress. Other: lettuce, sunflower seeds.

VITAMIN B$_2$ (RIBOFLAVIN)
WATER-SOLUBLE

SOME BENEFITS Essential for cell growth. Helps to maintain healthy mucous membranes, skin and eyes. Assists digestion. Needed for good eyesight, healthy skin and cellular growth. May help thyroid function

MAIN FOOD SOURCES Organ and muscle meats, wholegrains, milk, wheat germ, tofu, brewer's yeast, bran, eggs, cheese, yoghurt, green leafy vegetables, potatoes, tomatoes, almonds, sunflower seeds.

HERB SOURCES Very high: dandelion greens, watercress. Other: anise, lettuce, parsley, red clover, sage.

VITAMIN B$_3$ (NIACIN)
WATER-SOLUBLE

SOME BENEFITS May help brain function. Aids all aspects of digestion. Helps to lower blood cholesterol. Aids the release of energy from food. Improves blood circulation in the elderly. Has been used to treat schizophrenia. More than 1g of B$_3$ a day may result in unpleasant flushing and rashes of the skin.

MAIN FOOD SOURCES Organ and muscle meats, tofu, fish, brewer's yeast, wheat germ, nuts, bran, eggs, sunflower seeds, sprouted seeds and grains.

HERB SOURCES Very high: dandelion greens. High: landcress. Other: anise, catnep.

VITAMIN B$_5$ (PANTOTHENIC ACID)
WATER-SOLUBLE

Can cause diarrhoea if dose exceeds 10,000mg.

SOME BENEFITS Promotes health of adrenal glands. May help to prevent onset of premature baldness and ageing. Improves poor memory. Moderates allergic reactions.

MAIN FOOD SOURCES Organ meats, watermelon, mushrooms, salmon, egg yolks, peanuts, poultry, wholegrains, soya beans, sunflower and sesame seeds, sprouted seeds and grains.

HERB SOURCES Very high: dandelion leaf. High: nettle (young leaves). Other: catnep, mallow leaf, parsley, red clover, red raspberry, sage, thyme.

VITAMIN B$_6$
(PYRIDOXINE AND OTHERS)
WATER-SOLUBLE

Over 200mg daily can cause numbness in the hands and feet.

BENEFITS Protects against kidney stones, effects of radiation and x-rays. Protects mother and child from the effects of anaesthesia and helps to ease nausea in pregnancy.

REDUCED NIGHT CRAMPS Affects hair growth, colour and texture. May help to prevent dental decay and cancer. May help to ease PMS.

MAIN FOOD SOURCES Bran, wheat germ, brewer's yeast, organ and muscle meats, soya beans, fish, poultry, lentils and beans, avocado, sunflower seeds, peanuts, sprouted seeds and grains.

HERB SOURCES Very high: dandelion greens. Other: anise, catnep, mallow leaf, mullein, parsley, red clover, red raspberry, sage, thyme.

FOLIC ACID
(FOLACIN OR FOLATE)
WATER-SOLUBLE

BENEFITS Helps make antibodies. Needed for passing on hereditary characteristics. Used to treat schizophrenia. Essential for division of body cells. Important for making blood cells.

MAIN FOOD SOURCES Organ and muscle meats, chicken livers, dried yeast, dark green leafy vegetables, soya beans, wheat germ, wholegrains, kidney beans.

HERB SOURCES Red raspberry.

VITAMIN B$_{12}$
(CYANOCOBALAMIN)

Although water-soluble, this vitamin can be stored in the body. Vegan children are often deficient, as B$_{12}$ is found mainly in food of animal origin. Vegan adults don't seem to be as severely affected, as up to five years' store of B$_{12}$ may be kept in the body, and adults may also manufacture their own supply in the mouth or gastrointestinal tract.

BENEFITS Helps to form and regenerate red blood cells. Influences growth, fertility and resistance to infection. Helps to utilise fats, carbohydrates and protein.

MAIN FOOD SOURCES Liver and kidney, mushrooms, rabbit, milk, eggs, salmon and tuna, spirulina, some seaweeds, oysters.

HERB SOURCES Alfalfa, comfrey.

VITAMIN C
(ASCORBIC ACID)

Smokers may need to supplement.

WATER-SOLUBLE

BENEFITS Maintenance of healthy connective tissue and bone. Helps build resistance to infection, lowers blood cholesterol, reduces platelet stickiness. Important in production of proteins and hormones. Protects against stress; boosts the adrenals. Antioxidant properties may help to boost the immune system. Helps to heal the heart after heart attack; lowers blood pressure. Antibacterial, antiviral.

MAIN FOOD SOURCES All fruits, all vegetables.

HERB SOURCES Very high: alfalfa, dandelion greens, landcress, nettle, parsley, watercress. High: red clover. Other: catnep, calendula, cayenne, comfrey, garlic, oregano, paprika, peppermint, red raspberry, rosemary, sage, thyme, yarrow.

VITAMIN E
FAT-SOLUBLE

BENEFITS Antioxidant, reduces the cells' and heart's need for oxygen. Has been used to reduce angina pectoris symptoms and relieve heart conditions. Said to stimulate the immune system and alleviate allergic reactions. May help to prevent thrombosis.

MAIN FOOD SOURCES Wheat germ, bran and wheat cereals, wholegrains, parsley, broccoli, nuts, seeds, sprouting seeds and grains; wheat germ, sunflower, safflower, canola and olive oils.

HERB SOURCES Alfalfa, angelica, dandelion greens, garlic, landcress, nettle (young leaves), red raspberry, watercress, yarrow.

VITAMIN K
FAT-SOLUBLE

Large doses may cause haemolytic anaemia; it's not advised to take this vitamin as a supplement.

BENEFITS Essential for normal clotting of blood. Needed for the conversion of carbohydrates.

MAIN FOOD SOURCES Leafy green vegetables. Soya beans, peas, cauliflower, carrots, tomatoes, lean meat, liver.

MINERALS

CALCIUM

The body contains more calcium than any other mineral. Ninety-nine per cent is held in our teeth and bones. Weight-bearing exercise (such as walking) and vitamin D are essential for calcium and phosphorus to be absorbed into the body.

BENEFITS Relaxes nerves, induces sound sleep, decreases sensitivity to pain. Maintains a healthy heartbeat. Creates strong bones and teeth, helps to prevent osteoporosis. Helps to excrete blood fats from the body.

MAIN FOOD SOURCES Skimmed milk, milk, soya beans, yoghurt, cheese, almonds, sesame seeds, salmon, broccoli, eggs, fish and oysters.

HERB SOURCES Very high: watercress.
Other: alfalfa, angelica, anise, catnep, cayenne, comfrey, dandelion greens, garlic, mallow leaf, nettle (young leaves), parsley, red clover, red raspberry.

IRON

Iron is stored in the body. Women store less than men and need more because they lose it during menstruation. Weight loss diets are often deficient in sufficient iron. Children with learning or behavioural problems may be deficient.

Vegetarians need to be aware that iron absorption is impaired by whole grains, soya and other legumes. Vitamin C improves the absorption.

Tea or coffee drunk with meals or one hour before or after a meal inhibits absorption of iron.

BENEFITS Essential for oxygen transfer in the body. Helps the body resist disease. Prevents and cures iron-deficient anaemia. Helps muscles to function.

MAIN FOOD SOURCES There are two types of iron present in food: haeme iron and non-haeme iron. Haeme iron is found in meat (particularly organ meats), seafoods and poultry. Non-haeme iron is found in oats, lentils, broccoli, peas, salad vegetables, dried apricots and any foods which contain non-animal iron.

HERB SOURCES Very high: dandelion greens, landcress, nettle (young leaves), watercress. Other: anise, cayenne, chamomile, greens, garlic, mallow leaf, mullein, parsley, peppermint, red raspberry, rosemary, yarrow.

ZINC

More than 1–2 tablespoons of bran daily can reduce the absorption of zinc. Strict vegetarians or those with diets excessively high in fibre (mainly bran) may suffer from zinc deficiency.

Take on an empty stomach last thing at night when absorption isn't going to be interfered with.

BENEFITS May help decrease cholesterol deposits. Important in healing. Helps cure 'loss of taste'. Helps keep the prostate gland healthy. Helps to increase fertility.

MAIN FOOD SOURCES Beef, liver, lamb, chicken, nuts, seafood, beans, kidney, oats, bran, rice, wholemeal bread, yoghurt, cheese, milk.

HERB SOURCES Very high: dandelion greens.
Other: garlic, mallow leaf, nettle (young leaves), red raspberry, watercress.

The other major minerals are phosphorus, magnesium, potassium, sodium, chlorine, and sulphur. These are all found in the same foods as the minerals (calcium, iron, zinc) itemised above.

WATER

Our bodies are 76% water! In order to replace water lost through perspiration, digestive and excretory processes, we are urged to drink 6–8 glasses of water a day, but very little mention is made of the quality of the water. To drink this amount of chlorinated or soft water would be pretty damaging to our bodies.

Soft water is excellent for domestic use as it lathers easily but is not to be recommended for drinking. It is more acid than hard water and because of the acidity may have dissolved toxic trace elements like lead or cadmium from pipes and rocks. Soft water is also low in calcium, magnesium and trace elements. These elements are found in hard water and seem to give protection from cardiovascular disease.

A water purifier is a wise investment as not only does the water taste better but it also has chlorine and unwanted minerals removed.

SALT

Salt has always been an important commodity. The word 'salary' comes from the Latin *salarium* which was the money allowed to Roman soldiers for the purchase of salt.

Common salt is sodium chloride (40% sodium); it occurs in liquid form in lakes and the sea, and in rock form on land.

The amount of salt the body needs a day (between $\frac{1}{10}$th–$\frac{1}{5}$th of a teaspoon) is contained naturally in fish, meat, vegetables and grains. Yet on average we eat $1\frac{1}{2}$–2 or more teaspoons a day, in fast and convenience foods or added in cooking. If you consume a lot of salt you will need to wean yourself off it gradually.

Too much salt may result in fluid retention, over-loaded kidneys struggling to excrete the excess salt, circulatory problems and high blood pressure. In communities whose traditional diet does not include salt, high blood pressure is rare.

WAYS OF REDUCING SALT CONSUMPTION

- Slowly reduce the amount of salt you use in cooking. The family won't notice a gradual change but if you stop in one day they will.
- Try using more herbs in cooking.
- Stop putting the salt shaker on the table.
- Avoid salty foods such as crisps, pretzels etc.
- Avoid preserved meats and salami.
- Eat takeaway foods only occasionally.
- If you eat convenience and processed foods, buy only low-salt and salt-free varieties.

Nowadays it's possible to buy many low-salt or salt-free foods ranging from canned food, butter and margarine, bread, crackers, breakfast cereals and sauces. Low-salt products usually contain half to two-thirds less. When added to other dishes or used in sandwiches, the lack of salt isn't apparent.

Herb Salt

By using herbs in your cooking, you can increase the vitamin and mineral content; improve the flavour; and decrease the amount of salt by making use of the natural sodium found in herbs.

½ teacup sesame seeds
½ teacup yeast flakes
3–4 strips dried lemon peel, ground finely
3 tablespoons dried ground celery tops
1 teaspoon dried ground garlic
½ teaspoon dried ground dill seed
2 teacups dried ground parsley
2 teaspoons dried ground watercress
(if available)
1 teaspoon dried ground oregano
1 teaspoon dried ground lemon thyme
1 teaspoon ground coriander
1 teaspoon ground paprika
½ teaspoon ground black pepper

Grind the sesame seeds and yeast together. Add the remaining ingredients and mix well. Sieve and store in a jar in the refrigerator.

MAKES ABOUT 4 CUPS

FOOD ADDITIVES

On one hand we are pressured by advertising which presents convenience foods as being desirable and necessary to ensure the health, happiness and well-being of our families, attempting in a subtle way to make homemakers feel inadequate if they are not using these products. On the other hand we have the purists (often uninformed) who condemn all foodstuffs which are not in their original state. We need to decide in an educated way which, and how much (if any), convenience foods we are going to put on our plates.

To do this we need information, which these days is easy to obtain. Pamphlets on a variety of health topics can be obtained from the government health department.

Canned, frozen and packaged foods contain many chemicals to stabilise, add flavour and colour, modify texture, extend and preserve.

Preservatives are a necessary additive to many packaged foods to prevent contamination by bacteria, moulds and yeasts, many of which could cause illness or death. Yet because salt and sugar are cheap and such good preservatives, they are often added to foods in undesirable quantities.

(I have heard that corpses take longer to decompose these days due to the amount of preservatives in the bodies!)

The consumer is partly to blame for many of the other additives found in processed foods. In order to remain competitive, the manufacturer has to make the product appeal to the customer. Colour is added to make it look better; emulsifiers to prevent separation; thickeners to maintain consistency; mineral salts to enhance texture; bleaching agents to whiten foods; flavour enhancers to improve the taste. We get what we ask for and then grumble because we don't like the end result!

Not all additives are synthetic and, in fact, some of the natural additives (such as salt) are the most suspect in that they are dangerous to health if used excessively. Others, notably benzoic acid, carrageenan and tragacanth can create allergic reactions in sensitive people. Many food sensitivities may be traced to several additives (some synthetic colourings seem to be the particular culprits).

In the case of convenience foods, the food tends to get the blame but if eaten fresh might not cause a problem. For example, I have an innocuous-looking can of red beans on my desk as I write. The label states that the contents contain added sugar, salt and food acid. Now, when you cook a bean dish you sometimes add a little salt and almost never add sugar or food acid, so in the case of beans you have three ingredients which are unnecessary and, in the case of salt, harmful to your health.

A simple change would be to buy a bag of beans, put them to soak before you go to work and simmer them while you relax during the evening. Cool and pack them into suitable portions for future inclusion in recipes, pop them in the freezer, and you've made a considerable saving in cash outlay and salt and sugar intake.

I'm not saying that eating the can of beans is going to put you in hospital but the cumulative effect of these additives may be of concern if they form a large part of the daily dietary intake. Few of the additives have been tested long term so we have no way of knowing the eventual effects on our bodies of the increasing use of foods containing these chemicals. Let the buyer beware!

It is difficult for me to discuss food additives at length as it's beyond the scope of this book but it is one of the major nutritional issues of our time. If you are interested, I would urge you to read some or all of the books which I have listed in the Book List, in order that you can make informed choices. Some of these books tend to be biased one way or another but they are all good in their presentation of the facts and they enable us to weigh each fact against another and make choices.

THE BALANCED DIET

ACHIEVING THE BALANCED DIET, PAINLESSLY

We hear so much about the 'balanced diet' but even though there is plenty of literature available it's not always easy to translate this into the contents of the shopping trolley.

Let's try to get some sort of perspective as to how we can ensure that we and our families are having this 'balanced diet' without also having withdrawal symptoms and/or a nervous breakdown!

How many kilojoules (calories) a day? Men's and women's kilojoule (calorie) needs differ.

The average daily kilojoule (calorie) expenditure for men is 8200–16,400 kJ (1960–3920 cals) depending on height and type of work/activity.

For women the average daily kilojoule (calorie) expenditure is 6500–12,300 kJ (1550–2935 cals), again depending on height and type of work and activity. (If the kilojoules confuse you they may be converted to calories by dividing by 4.2.)

WHERE ARE HEALTHY KILOJOULES FOUND?

The following is a daily plan for an 'average' woman about 35 years old, 168cm (5ft 6in) tall, weighing 58–65kg (128–143lb), and moderately active. She would possibly need 7000–8000 kJ (1670–1910 cals) a day.

(a) BREADS, CEREALS AND STARCHY VEGETABLES: 6 SERVES

Six serves means a total of: 2 slices bread + 1 serving (30g/1oz) breakfast cereal + 1 cup cooked pasta + 1 medium potato + $\frac{1}{2}$ cup pumpkin + $\frac{1}{2}$ cup cooked corn kernels or peas. Total: approx. 3055 kJ (730 cals) You can juggle these around if you like, as long as the kilojoules (calories) remain the same.

(b) FRUIT: 3 SERVES

Three serves of fruit means 1 medium apple, 1 orange and 1 pear or their equivalent in weight or size. Total: approx. 900 kJ (215 cals).

(c) VEGETABLES: 3 SERVES

Three serves of vegetables means 3 cups after cooking. Total: approx. 600 kJ (145 cals). Be aware that 1 medium avocado has 1607 kJ (385 cals)! I use it instead of butter on toast so a little goes a long way. Peas also have a higher kilojoule value than most vegetables but are high in fibre so should be included. Try to buy a wide variety of different-coloured fruit and vegetables in order to get the broadest range of vitamins and minerals. Steaming, pressure cooking or microwaving preserves the greatest number of vitamins.

(d) MEAT, FISH AND LEGUMES

125g (4oz) lean meat + 60g (2oz) tuna or 200g ($6\frac{1}{2}$oz) fish or 2 eggs and 80g (3oz) meat + 30g (1oz) nuts. Total: approx. 1600 kJ (380 cals) (based on fillet steak which has more kilojoules (calories) than most fish).

Or 250g (8oz) tofu or tempeh + 2 eggs + 10 almonds. Total: approx. 1700 kJ (405 cals).

(e) MILK AND MILK PRODUCTS

$1\frac{1}{4}$ cups (300ml/10fl oz) daily as skim milk or yoghurt or $\frac{3}{4}$ cup (90g/3oz) cottage cheese or 40g ($1\frac{1}{3}$oz) hard cheese such as cheddar. Total: approx. 369 kJ (90 cals). You can mix these any way you like as long as the total amounts remain the same. Be aware that cottage cheese is a very poor source of calcium.

(f) FATS AND OILS.

The total allowance for the day of butter/margarine or cooking oils or cream/sour cream is 1 tablespoon, which is approx. 615 kJ (145 cals). Not much is it? 1 teaspoon low-oil mayonnaise is 52 kJ (12 cals).

(g) WATER

Every day have 6–8 glasses of water. If your tap water is chlorinated you would be wise to buy a filter or purifier as this amount of chlorinated water could be doing you more harm than good.

Fresh foods make an important part of the balanced diet

(h) EXTRAS

1 tablespoon sugar in tea or coffee during the day 286 kJ (68 cals) + 1 teaspoon marmalade 55 kJ (13 cals) + glass white wine 463 kJ (110 cals). This leaves approx. 57 kJ (14 cals) which could be accounted for by eating a fraction more of any of the food groups above.

Try not to have more than 3 cups of ordinary tea or coffee in a day. Avoid drinking tea or coffee for an hour before or after a meal, as 65% of the usable iron content of your meal will be destroyed!

BE AWARE OF THESE KILOJOULES (CALORIES)!

1 serve chicken and chips	2812 kJ (670 cals)
1 hamburger	2341 kJ (560 cals)
1 thick shake	1226 kJ (292 cals)
½ regular thin pizza	1775 kJ (423 cals)
1 x 11cm (4½in) meat pie	2123 kJ (507 cals)
1 serve fish and chips	2296 kJ (548 cals)
1 croissant	1000 kJ (235 cals)

'LITTLE' EXTRAS

Snacks such as the ones listed below are really 'non-food' in that they are loaded with fat or sugar, are easy, quick, and appealing to eat or drink and are usually eaten between or after meals—particularly during the evening when watching television or socialising. It would be very easy to consume your whole daily allowance of kilojoules (calories) in one evening of watching a video or talking with friends!

small serve cheese and biscuits	600 kJ (143 cals)
100g (3⅓oz) white chocolate	522 kJ (125 cals)
100g (3⅓oz) milk chocolate	526 kJ (125 cals)
small packet potato crisps	134 kJ (32 cals)
60g (2oz) salted peanuts	348 kJ (83 cals)
25g (1oz) corn chips	120 kJ (28 cals)
1 middy of beer	467 kJ (110 cals)
30ml (1fl oz) liqueur	439 kJ (104 cals)
1 glass sherry	360 kJ (85 cals)
1 glass wine, dry	328 kJ (78 cals)
1 glass wine, sweet	463 kJ (110 cals)

Now, having thoroughly depressed you with these horrible statistics I would hasten to add that I am not a purist and certainly wouldn't suggest that anyone else should be. I enjoy chocolate, rich desserts and the occasional glass of wine but I don't treat them as a daily necessity and am aware that I might need to eat fewer kilojoules (calories) the following day to 'balance the binge' as I put on weight very easily.

Total deprivation of foods which you crave is dangerous as it can lead to excesses when the urge finally gets the better of you! Let's not forget that 'a little of what you fancy does you good'!

High kilojoule (calorie), high 'saturated fat' or sugary foods which are often low in vitamins, minerals, complex carbohydrates and fibre may be treated as occasional indulgences.

Even if you don't put on weight the fat may be working away silently, clogging your arteries and making sure that the heart attack or stroke happens.

SUBSTITUTIONS FOR A BALANCED DIET

➤ Avoid fatty cuts of meat, especially luncheon meats, sausages, salami and chicken skin. Substitute with skinless chicken, turkey, tofu, tempeh, lean cuts of meat.

➤ Avoid whole milk and whole milk products. Substitute with skim or low-fat milk and yoghurt.

➤ Use small portions only of high-fat cheeses such as cheddar, Parmesan, Jarlsberg. Substitute with ricotta, cottage cheese, Edam. Choose reduced-fat Cheddars.

➤ When a recipe uses a stock cube, the salt may be omitted.

➤ If there is bacon in a recipe it should be trimmed of all fat.

➤ Invest in a non-stick pan with a lid. You will be able to fry onions and mushrooms in a little water instead of oil.

➤ If a savoury recipe calls for cream you can almost always substitute some or all with yoghurt. Mix a little cornflour into the yoghurt before adding to the pan. This will prevent yoghurt curdling.

➤ Mix mayonnaise half and half with low-fat yoghurt to drastically reduce the kilojoules (calories).

➤ A delicious 'jam' may be made by soaking dried apricots overnight in water to cover and then blending with lemon juice and honey to taste. This jam only keeps for about a week in the refrigerator but contains much healthier ingredients than ordinary jam which is 50% white sugar.

➤ Use egg whites instead of whole egg to coat chicken pieces etc. If a recipe calls for several eggs you can substitute 2 egg whites for 1 whole egg, thus saving kilojoules (calories) and cholesterol.

➤ 'Sneak feed' the children by mixing finely grated carrot into the peanut butter or spread for their sandwiches.

➤ Don't butter the bread if you are using cottage cheese, peanut butter or spread or other fillings with similar textures. No-one will ever know!

➤ Don't use butter straight from the fridge for spreading on sandwiches—you'll use twice as much as you need.

➤ Marinate meat before grilling. The marinade will keep the meat juicy and can be used to baste during cooking.

Finally, remember that exercise is equally as important as diet. Regular exercise stimulates the metabolic rate (which slows down dramatically if you reduce your kilojoule (calorie) intake and don't exercise). I find that a 30 minute walk in the evening about half an hour after dinner makes me feel really good about myself and my body. Choose the same time of day if possible so that a habit is formed.

The older you are, the more important exercise becomes. Your metabolic rate slows down as you get older and you need fewer kilojoules (calories) to maintain your correct weight. Weight-bearing exercise such as walking is also needed to help prevent osteoporosis in ageing bones.

CHAPTER EIGHT

STRESS, EXERCISE, RELAXATION AND MEDITATION

This chapter is about stress, exercise, relaxation and

meditation, and the part they play in our appearance, health

and contentment. No amount of cosmetic attention will make

us look good if we are stressed, unhealthy and/or unhappy.

Good health shows in bright eyes, shiny hair, clear

unblemished skin, firm muscles and a positive,

vibrant outlook on life.

Flowers by Lisa Milasas

STRESS

There are two types of stress:

➤ eustress, which is the healthy stress which we need in order to function in everyday life; and

➤ dystress, which is the unhealthy, unresolved stress that is emotionally and physically damaging.

To understand the difference in the two types of stress we need to know a little of what happens to our bodies in a stressful situation. Here is one scene, typical of a eustress situation:

You are walking down a busy street when you see a car completely out of control heading for a small child standing on the footpath a little way from you.

The shock of the situation causes the hypothalamus, deep in your brain, to release substances to the pituitary (which is below the hypothalamus and attached by a stalk); the hormones released by the pituitary race through the blood to the adrenal glands which are situated on top of the kidneys; adrenalin hormones are pumped out into the bloodstream, causing the blood pressure to rise and the heart to beat faster; your digestion comes to a standstill and your blood-sugar level rises to give energy to muscles. These changes happen so quickly that you are instantly mobilised to do a fast sprint (which would normally be beyond you), scoop the child into your arms (plus your briefcase and/or shopping and laundry) and get out of harm's way before the car hits the spot. The car's driver is unhurt, the child is safe, and you are triumphant and happy.

Other changes now take place in your body, to return it to its normal, relaxed state:

The excess blood sugar is regulated by a surge of insulin produced by the pancreas; heartbeat returns to normal; digestion begins again; the liver begins a 'mopping up' operation of surplus hormones and the acid in the muscles is neutralised. You can now hand the child back to a tearful, thankful mother and go home to your family feeling like a heroic character from a fiction novel!

Eustress is exhilarating and can add sparkle to our lives; it can stimulate our alertness and abilities. We have all experienced the all-out effort of competition; the dry mouth and sweating palms before going on stage, making a speech or sitting an exam; the heady thrill of watching a race when your child is coming in first, of plucking up courage to ask for a raise (and getting it)—these stresses are healthy. They have a beginning and a satisfactory end in which the body returns to its normal and relaxed state.

If the stress is ongoing and can't be resolved as satisfactorily and quickly as the one in my story, it becomes a dystress situation. The possibility of developing physical and emotional illness is very real as the body doesn't receive the signals to reverse the chemical process and you are in a constant state of 'flight or fight'. The adrenalin, hormones, sugar, lactic acid and urine are retained instead of being dispersed. Some of the problems which may arise are high blood pressure, angina, coronary thrombosis, excess cholesterol, stomach ulcers, colitis, cancer, migraine, back problems, atherosclerosis, depression and nervous breakdown.

There are many stresses which continue day after day and which often don't have an obvious solution or which have a solution which is so unpleasant that we choose to live with the unhealthy situation.

Some of these stresses may be: loss or possible loss of a job; loss of a loved one; partner problems; your children out of control and getting into trouble; too heavy workload with no end in sight; friction with workmates or neighbours; chronic shortage of money; and loneliness.

These distressing problems need to be resolved for the sake of our health. Counsellors who are trained and willing to help are available in most towns.

Dystress includes 'chemical' stress, a by-product of the enormous technological changes which have occurred in the last fifty years. We have synthetic materials, artificial fertilisers and pesticides, antibiotics, traffic fumes, television, and additives to processed foods.

Humans are very adaptable but these changes have happened so quickly that we are finding more and more people are developing chemical stress. Migraines, allergic reactions, asthma and many other diseases are a result of the body's inability to cope with chemical stress.

The warning signs of stress include:

- Backache
- Diarrhoea
- Disturbed sleep or insomnia
- Frequent infections
- Indigestion
- Irritability
- Poor concentration
- Problems with family and/or workmates
- Restlessness
- Sadness and/or tearfulness
- Tense, sore muscles
- Withdrawal
- Worry

COPING WITH STRESS

If we are to help our bodies cope with unhealthy dystress, we need to learn to like ourselves, find methods of defusing stressful situations, make sure that we are eating the right food, take time to do the things we enjoy, learn to share our feelings, take adequate exercise, get enough rest and sleep, and learn to meditate.

LEARNING TO LIKE OURSELVES

The messages we receive from other people and from the television, radio and newspapers are largely negative. It seems that 'bad news is good news'. If we admire some aspect of ourselves we are seen to be conceited. If we say negative things about ourselves, people will console us. From childhood we are rewarded for misery; we are offered sweets or cuddles for being unhappy. How often are we rewarded for our laughter and happiness?

Begin to make a conscious effort towards positivity. Don't get drawn into other people's or your own misery; give the bad news a miss. Avoid being in the company of complainers. Catch yourself if you are whingeing and STOP—your stress levels will benefit immediately.

I have a daughter who is the 'Pollyanna' of our family. If the roof caved in she would probably gaze up and say 'What a wonderful view of the sky'! She has had more than her share of woe during her lifetime but has realised that dwelling on it doesn't improve the situation—quite the reverse. She is not pious, just positive. We all can make a deliberate choice between being negative or positive, happy or unhappy.

You are unique.
There is no-one like you in the whole world.
Enjoy and cherish the feeling that
you are special.
Remember your successes when you are
feeling defeated.

FINDING METHODS OF DEFUSING STRESSFUL SITUATIONS

If you experience problems when dealing with people, you would probably benefit from one of the many courses which are available these days. Assertiveness training is a good one for people who are either too aggressive or too passive. We tend to either get angry or to 'give in' in a confrontational situation. Assertiveness training teaches us to have the courage to state what we want and how we feel but also to listen to the other person's point of view.

Learn to be flexible. You may be over-rigid in your views; things don't always have to be done your way; people are entitled to think differently to you. The tree that bends before the wind survives; the one which stays unbending breaks.

EATING THE RIGHT FOOD

We know that in order to get peak performance from our car we have to care for it; the body needs cleaning and waxing and the engine requires good quality oil and fuel. The car will run on cheap fuel but the engine will wear out more quickly and the daily performance will be poor. We often don't treat our bodies with the same consideration.

Recent statistics show that three out of five meals eaten in Australia today are 'takeaway' foods which are frequently high in fat and low in vitamins, minerals and fibre.

Unless we treat our bodies with at least as much respect as our vehicles our performance will suffer and our engine and chassis will wear out quickly! (For a more detailed discussion on food, see Chapter Seven.)

TAKING TIME TO DO THE THINGS WE ENJOY

If you feel tired and jaded with little enthusiasm for life, maybe you aren't making time for fun. It's very easy to slip into a grinding routine to 'get up, go to work, come home, more work, go to bed'.

Leisure time is vital in order to keep enthusiasm for the other aspects of our lives. We have a right to this free time but often feel guilty about taking it. Work off tensions by gardening, pursuing a hobby, or by joining a club.

Take time to be alone, doing nothing. There is a profound difference between doing something positive and just creating 'busyness'. We are told as children 'don't just sit there, do something'; change this to 'don't do something, just sit there'!

Burnout is a mental, physical and emotional condition which is often not recognised until we are in real danger; it is often the result of 'all work, no play'. These are some of the symptoms:

- being permanently tired
- having no enthusiasm for work, family or friends
- finding it difficult to laugh and getting upset very easily

- having a feeling of 'impending doom' hanging over you
- suffering from backaches, headaches and stomach aches
- inability to sleep; or waking up in the morning feeling anxious and as tired as when you went to bed.

If some or all of the above apply, then you may be suffering from burnout. The suggestions in this book regarding exercise, leisure, food and meditation may be helpful but you may also need to get professional help from a trained counsellor.

LEARNING TO SHARE OUR FEELINGS

Find someone with whom you can share your feelings. Don't keep a 'stiff upper lip'—crying is a great tension reliever. Stretch your arms out wide and laugh often; this has been found to disperse stress and strengthen the autoimmune system!

TAKING ADEQUATE EXERCISE

Research shows that physical exercise is the best tension reliever. If you arrive home from work with a tension headache and a stiff neck, a long bath or reading a book on your bed will slowly disperse the tension but a brisk walk, game of squash or something similarly active would achieve the same result much more quickly.

On the rare occasions that my mother was angry she scrubbed floors ferociously. I don't think she deliberately chose to scrub floors as a therapy but subconsciously she must have known that what she was doing was a great 'defuser'. My father and I always kept out of her way until the scrubbing was done and Mum was restored to her normal good humour.

Problems always seem less important when you are walking, swimming, running, cycling, or are involved in any other physical pursuits, and apart from the mental benefits, physical exercise uses up excess adrenalin.

Take time out to do gardening—a
relaxing way to work off tensions

GETTING ENOUGH REST AND SLEEP

Our bodies need six to eight hours of uninterrupted sleep in order to renew cells and restore our nervous system. If we are deprived of sufficient sleep we become irritable and low in energy and our brains refuse to function adequately. Externally, skin becomes sallow and we develop dark circles and 'bags' under the eyes.

LEARNING TO MEDITATE

Meditation is a wonderful 'de-stressor'. After you have been doing it for a while and your stress is under control, you will find that your meditation will deepen and become more spiritual. (More on meditation later in this chapter.)

EXERCISE

'The longest journey starts with just one step.'
—THE TAO TE CHING (5TH CENTURY BC)

Exercise gives improved heart, lung and circulation function, more flexible joints, and stronger muscles and bones. The appearance of skin and hair will improve and sleep will be of a better quality. Stress levels and blood pressure will be reduced and tempers will become sweeter.

The most difficult part of beginning any exercise programme is making the commitment to do it and then putting on your walking shoes and stepping out of the door or dragging your swimsuit out of mothballs and heading off to the beach or pool. If you are overweight or underfit a dreadful lethargy sets in. A picture of months of deprivation and hard work forms in your mind and you decide that it's easier to stay as you are. Exercise will help you feel more in control of your life, and this leads to an improved self-image.

Advances in technology mean that we are becoming far more sedentary and the advent of computers, television sets and video machines means that our leisure time is more passive than ever before. Our bodies are made to be active. We need to stretch, walk, run, lift and carry but because of the inactive lives we lead, joints become stiff, muscles and ligaments weak and these normal activities often lead to strained, pulled muscles and back problems. Our bodies lose that vital look and appear flabby and soft.

The last ten years has seen a huge explosion of interest in exercise—it is the fashionable thing to do. Unfortunately, the videos and magazines usually feature slim, athletic, sexy young women and bronzed, athletic, sexy young men with glistening muscles to promote and demonstrate their programmes. These types of programmes exclude more people than they include, as most of us can't identify with these rare and unlikely role models.

Aim to maximise your own potential and appearance. Create a mental picture of how you want to be and see yourself looking and being like that right now. This technique works really well as it creates a feeling of confidence which is vital to well-being and to the continuation of any self-improvement programme.

If surplus body weight is a problem, the extra kilojoules (calories) lost during exercise will help to give a healthy, slim body. If we sit around feeling fat, hungry and sorry for ourselves we use only 100 kJ (24 cals) in fifteen minutes. A brisk walk would burn about 315 kJ (75 cals) in the same amount of time, take the mind off food and leave us feeling great!

Cycling and walking are excellent forms of exercise

It is a proven fact that unless people who have been on a weight loss programme increase their metabolic rate by exercising, they may have to stay on a low kilojoule (calorie) intake for the rest of their lives as their metabolic rate may have dropped during the dieting process. What a grim prospect!

The vital thing is to enjoy the exercise which you have chosen to do. There is no benefit to be gained, either physical or emotional, by torturing yourself, as you would then begin to find reasons for not continuing.

I dislike regimented exercise intensely—not for me the strict regime of morning and evening exercise work-outs—but as I am a Taurean who loves food and who tastes food all the time when I am cooking (which is very often), my weight balloons up and down if not kept in some sort of gentle check. My preferred exercises are gardening, walking, using a mini-trampoline and stretching using the 'Yoga Salute to the Sun' (this chapter). The latter keeps me supple as I would otherwise get very stiff from spending many hours a day at a computer.

Here are some ways of exercising which might inspire you when you see the kilojoules (calories) losses! (A table of kilojoules (calories) expended during various activities is given later in this chapter.)

WALKING

*When I am alone, as it were,
completely myself...
walking after a good meal...
ideas flow best and most abundantly.
Whence and how they come, I know not;
nor can I force them.*
—**WOLFGANG AMADEUS MOZART
(1756–1791)**

We have been walking since we were about one year old and it is so familiar to us that it's often not perceived as being exercise. We don't have to learn to do it, we don't need to buy special clothes (but a comfortable pair of shoes is essential), we don't have to drive anywhere. We just walk out of our homes, round a block or two and there you are—painlessly, pleasurably exercised. It can also be very precious time in which a family can be together, sharing the pleasure of each other's company. Less and less time is being spent in family communication.

Research shows that walking is the most beneficial exercise of all and it also has a bonus of being a great problem-solving time. If I have a problem I save it until my walk time; it feels less important out of doors and it is often solved by the time I am back at my front door.

To gain the maximum benefit with no pain (thank goodness, the 'no pain, no gain' school of thought has now been largely de-bunked), begin at a slow walk for about 2–3 minutes, steam up for about 12 minutes, walk moderately for 4 minutes, steam up until you are about 3 minutes from home and slow down to a contented amble. When you are much fitter you can miss the middle 'moderate' bit. You should arrive home feeling smug and healthy. It's important to plan a route where you aren't going to have to continually stop for road crossings or a lot of the benefit will be lost.

CYCLING

If cycling appeals to you, try to plan a route where you will be able to cycle at a steady speed without having to slow down for too many traffic crossings or spend the time breathing diesel or petrol fumes. As with walking, it's good to begin your ride slowly, speed up and slow down again a few minutes from home—this gives muscles a chance to warm up and cool down.

SWIMMING

Excellent for toning muscles, improving circulation and lung capacity. An easy way of exercising for the overweight as the water gives support and the joints don't become stressed. Swimming is not so good if you are staving off osteoporosis as only weight bearing exercise such as walking and skipping are useful for strengthening bones.

SKIPPING

'Easy does it.' (If you are elderly, unfit or overweight don't even try it.) Start with 1–2 minutes and increase as you lose the grams (ounces).

As skipping is quite hard work it's a good idea to mix it with other, less demanding exercise.

WALKING UPSTAIRS

If you have stairs in your house you can lose a lot of weight walking up and down them, and that loss can be doubled if you carry a 6kg (12lb) weight. If you are overweight you will lose more; if average weight, less. This is another exercise to avoid if you are very overweight or unfit.

DANCING

Put a rock-and-roll music CD or cassette into your player and DANCE—just let yourself go with the music. Depending on how outrageously wild you get, you will lose a lot of kilojoules (calories) and it's one of the most energy-raising, fun and healthy things you can do.

If none of these exercise suggestions appeals to you, or if you like the idea of more structured exercise programmes, there are many good books devoted to the subject, and most towns conduct yoga, swimming, aerobic or other types of classes.

Most sports are good energy burners but the disadvantage can be that they are often played only once a week. It's much better to spend 30 minutes a day regularly than to do a potentially stressful and exhausting 2–2½ hours 1 day a week. We often read about the person who drives to work, sits at a desk, drives home, has a smoke, has a drink and drops dead after a game of tennis at the weekend! Whatever exercise you decide to do don't let it become a burden or a competitive chore. Enjoy it.

YOGA SALUTE TO THE SUN

This is a deeply relaxing, active meditation technique which I chose to include in the exercise section because of its beneficial effects on the body. It reduces stomach fat; stretches muscles and ligaments, bringing flexibility to the spine and limbs; and increases breathing capacity.

This exercise is a boon to those who have been inactive and want to restore flexibility to their bodies in a gentle way. Done each day for 15–20 minutes, this exercise will make your body stronger and more supple. Do it out of doors if possible, facing the rising sun, but if the weather isn't good enough it can be done in front of an open window.

Don't force anything. As you loosen up, the exercise will become progressively easier, but until then just allow the body to do the best it can.

Keep the breathing and movements slow and gentle to allow muscles and tendons time to adapt.

STEPS 1–3

1   *Stand straight with your feet shoulder-width apart. Inhale deeply but gently and slowly, and visualise the sun beginning to rise.*

2   *As you exhale, bring your palms together in front of your chest in a prayer position.*

3   *Inhale slowly and simultaneously stretch your arms overhead, tilt your pelvis slightly forward and look up at your hands.*

STEPS 4–5

4   *Exhale as you bend slowly from the waist until you are touching the floor in front of your feet. (Until this is easy, just bend as far as you can, flexing the knees slightly.)*

5   *Inhale slowly as you lower into a squat, bending your left knee to a right angle and stepping back on the right foot. Turn the toes of your right foot back and straighten your body from the top of your head to the heel.*

STEP 6

Hold your breath and step your left foot back next to your right foot so that your body is in a 'push up' position.

STEP 7

Exhale slowly as you drop your knees to the floor and stick your bottom up in the air. Bend your elbows until your chin and chest rest on the floor. Continuing to exhale, lower your body to the floor. Straighten your legs but keep your toes curled back.

STEP 8

Inhale as you push down on your hands. Slowly lift your head and gently straighten your elbows (as much as you can without straining the lower back). Arch slowly upwards until you are looking straight ahead, keeping your pelvis on the ground.

STEP 9

As you exhale, lift your buttock all the way up in the air and put your head down so that you form a triangle with the floor. Hold for 10 seconds.

STEP 10

Inhale, bend your right knee and step your right foot forwards between your hands.

STEPS 11–12

11 *As you exhale, keeping your hands as near to the floor as possible, straighten your right leg and bring your left one forward next to it.*

12 *Inhale while slowly enrolling your spine, lifting your head last. Raise your head, lift your arms high on either side of your head and visualise the sun rising again.*

STEP 13

As you exhale let your arms slowly come down to your sides. Stand quietly for a moment or two feeling the power of the rising sun filling you with energy and positivity. Enjoy!

AVERAGE KILOJOULES (CALORIES) EXPENDED DURING EXERCISE

It's impossible to give completely accurate figures in this chart as many different factors are involved—it's an inspiring guide, none the less.

ACTIVITY	KILOJOULES USED PER HOUR	ACTIVITY	KILOJOULES USED PER HOUR
Sleeping	300 (72 cals)	Skating	1490 (355 cals)
Watching TV	400 (95 cals)	Dancing rock-and-roll	1500 (358 cals)
Typing	500 (120 cals)	Cycling quite fast	1680 (400 cals)
Cooking	525 (125 cals)	Walking quite fast	1690 (403 cals)
Ironing	630 (150 cals)	Swimming	1830 (437 cals)
Walking slowly	735 (175 cals)	Heavy gardening	1890 (450 cals)
Croquet	735 (175 cals)	Walking upstairs	1890 (450 cals)
Cricket	735 (175 cals)	Energetic skipping	2520 (602 cals)
Light gardening	1000 (238 cals)	Power walking	2940 (702 cals)
Badminton	1130 (270 cals)	Running	3100 (740 cals)
Moderate cycling	1260 (300 cals)	Squash	3100 (740 cals)
Walking quite fast	1260 (300 cals)	Walking upstairs	3530 (843 cals)
Tennis	1470 (350 cals)	carrying 6kg	
Gentle jogging	1480 (353 cals)	(12lb)weight	

RELAXATION

Without relaxation, meditation is not possible.

Devote the first few minutes of each meditation time to relaxation. First the breathing. This breathing may release deep-seated sadness, anger or other emotions. Allow these emotions to surface, cry, be angry—whatever happens is fine.

Take each breath slowly and gently into the dark, secret place deep within you where you feel at peace.

As you release the breath, release any fear, hostility, anger or sadness. Experience the feelings flowing out with each breath.

Keep the breathing relaxed and easy, taking peace and tranquillity into your body and releasing negativity as the breath flows out.

Now that you have relaxed your mind, you are ready to begin relaxing your body. Do all the movements and breathing very gently and slowly.

At first the breathing and relaxation may take up most of your allotted meditation time. Don't worry—this is needed until you are practised in this technique. After a while you will be able to relax by breathing deeply and taking your awareness around your body, breathing tensions out with the breath—anywhere, any time.

When practising this relaxation, breathe in slowly through your nose and out through your mouth in a gentle sigh…aaaaaaaahhhhhh.

The first time you practise this technique, it's easier if a friend or partner reads it to you in a quiet, slow voice.

Take your awareness to your feet. As you inhale, tense your feet by curling your toes. Hold. As you exhale, uncurl. Feel the difference.

Now, move the attention to your lower legs. As you gently inhale, tighten the calves, hold for a few seconds. As you breathe out, let the tension go.

Tense your thighs as you breathe in…hold… and as you breathe out, relax, let the tension flow out like thick oil. Your legs feel heavy and relaxed.

As you gently and deeply breathe in, take your awareness to your buttock, stomach and genitals, tense and hold for a few seconds. Let the tension flow away as you breathe out. From the waist down, you feel as heavy as lead…soft and relaxed.

Lift your shoulders towards your ears as you breath in…hold it…feel the tension flow away as you breathe out.

Tense your chest and arch your spine as you breathe in…hold it…breathe out the tension and r e l a x.

Let your awareness flow to your hands. As you breathe in, tighten them into fists, straighten your arms until the elbows are locked, feel the tension from your hands to your shoulders, hold it. As the breath flows out of your body, let the tension flow from your arms and hands, let your arms and hands flop…heavy…limp…relaxed.

Your whole body, from your neck down, is relaxed…calm…comfortable.

As you breathe deeply in and out, let your head roll gently from one side to the other, feel the tension drain from your neck… Do a few times.

Your awareness is now in your head. Inhale as you clench your teeth and squeeze your mouth into a tight little purse…hold it…and relax as the breath leaves you.

As you breathe in, open your mouth wide…yawn…and relax as you breathe out. Leave your lips together but the teeth slightly apart and your jaw relaxed.

Breathe in as you squeeze your mouth, eyes, ears and skin on your skull tight and wrinkle your nose upwards…hold…breathe out and relax…let the tensions drain away…feel the difference…

Let your attention roam gently over your body, beginning at the feet. If any tension has returned, breathe into it and release all the tension with your out breath.

Feel the freedom…feel the peace…enjoy the feeling. As you exhale, feel the relaxation. Let your mind drift and float free. If thoughts come, be gentle with them, move them to one side until later.

When you are ready to return, count slowly backwards from ten to one. When you have reached one you will feel rested, calm and alert. If you wish to sleep, omit the counting. Your sleep will be deep and refreshing.

MEDITATION

Anyone can meditate. You already meditate. It doesn't require special esoteric training or mysterious secret mantras but it does require time and patience.

All of us have learned several skills in our lives, such as how to walk and talk; cook; ride a bicycle; drive a car; operate a computer; take care of a family; earn a salary; learn to play a guitar or to speak Japanese. So many things, all so difficult and requiring time and patience, but once mastered, able to be done intuitively.

Think about driving a car. When you began you had to remember so much: look in the mirrors; use the clutch to change gears; ease off the clutch to use the accelerator; steering and on and on and on. You now get into the car and drive away using an instinctive series of actions which has become part of your deep understanding.

Put simplistically, meditation is the art of doing one thing at a time. You meditate if you stop what you are doing and just 'be'. At first the process of 'stopping' will feel as difficult as learning any other skill, but slowly it will happen and you will begin to experience positive changes happening in your life.

You meditate constantly without being aware that you are doing it. You are meditating when you silently, mindlessly, watch the flames in a fire. When you are alone with your mind drifting, not thinking, you are meditating. Whenever you are totally immersed in an experience in which time stands still and thought processes stop, you are meditating.

When you are walking, running, swimming, dancing or juggling for a long time, the thought process stops and you become the running, not the runner, the dancing not the dancer, the walking not the walker. Thought stops and there is just the running or the walking or the dancing.

Babies meditate all the time—watch them when they think they are alone. They haven't yet learnt to 'fill in time'; they are content just to 'be'.

You are starting on an journey of discovery where the only thing to expect is the unexpected.

Your mind is tricky; it will resent meditation and will fight to fill your mind. It's very good at 'chattering'; it's been doing it for many years and won't see any good reason for stopping. Be gentle with it. When thoughts come, move them to one side, tell them 'later' and return to meditation. At first you will have to do this every few seconds. Don't give up, don't feel a failure; this is new to both you and your brain, and you will need patience.

The idea is implanted during our childhood that in order to win approval from other humans we have to be logical, useful, and busy. We spend our lives trying to please others and in the process we lose sight of who we are.

If we spend all our waking hours with other people or fully occupied with work, we allow no time to 'be with ourselves'. Unless we spend time in silence, experiencing our aloneness and uniqueness, our brains remain like a cluttered attic full of our own and other people's junk.

Begin today by throwing that junk away and experiencing the freedom which comes from meditation. It won't happen overnight—it took time to learn to play the guitar or speak Japanese and it will take time to re-learn to meditate. The benefits will be enormous on both a physical and spiritual level.

You will: find some answers to the questions 'Who am I?'; feel more in touch with the Universe and everyone in it; gain intuitive knowledge and inner understanding; be more at peace and less stressed; be more effective in your work; and lose your feelings of loneliness and replace them with a sense of 'aloneness'.

*Sitting silently on a beach watching the sun
begin to set, hearing the 'shhhoosh' of the
waves on the shore, feeling the breeze as it
touches your face, is a meditation.
Seeing the changing colours, with your heart
and not your mind.
Hearing the sounds of the ocean, with your
heart and not your ears, is a meditation.
Feeling the breeze without thinking.
You and the sunset, the beach, the ocean,
the wind become one.
The problems cease to exist. The striving
ceases to exist. The stress ceases to exist. You
become one with the moment.*

Most of the time we can't sit on a beach and meditate so we need to find simple ways to reach the same 'no-mind' space. We need to drop the idea of hard work; meditation is 'sitting silently, doing nothing'. Words such as 'trying', 'working at it', 'failure' have no place in meditation.

FIRST STEPS TO MEDITATION

All we need to meditate is a time and a place where we will know that we are alone. The best times are early morning and last thing at night. The place can be a corner of your bedroom, the garden shed or anywhere private.

Make your meditation place (no matter how small) a sanctuary and decorate it with something which gives you pleasure and calms you, such as a piece of driftwood, a crystal, a beautiful stone, a flower. Burn some incense if it pleases you. Wear soft, loose comfortable clothing and have a chair, cushion or meditation stool to sit on.

Whenever you are meditating or relaxing, rest your hands, palms up, on your knees and put the thumb and second finger together very lightly. This is called the 'Relaxation Response', your mind will recognise this as a signal to relax.

If you make these small rituals your mind will come to accept that in this place, at this time, we meditate. Later on you will be able to meditate anywhere, any time.

From the four choices below, find a comfortable way to sit or lie. If you choose to sit, you need to sit straight—imagine a line from the top of your head to the base of your spine.

1 You can sit on a straight-backed chair with your feet firmly on the floor and a little apart and your hands resting softly on your knees, palms up, second finger and thumb lightly together.
2 Or use a cushion on the floor…or sit with your back against a wall. Your legs should be folded and crossed but if this is uncomfortable they may be straight with a cushion under the knees to prevent stress. Hands resting on your knees, palms up, second finger and thumb together.
3 Meditation stools are available now and they are low timber seats which you sit on with your legs underneath (as in the picture at right). The angle of the seat makes sitting straight easy. Have your hands resting on your knees, palms up, second finger and thumb lightly together.
4 You can lie down with a small pillow under your head and another under your knees. (It's very easy to go to sleep like this though!) Hands resting loosely by your sides, palms up, second finger and thumb lightly together.

Whichever position you choose is all right; there is no 'right' or 'wrong'.

Sit or lie quietly for a few moments, hearing sounds far away, not analysing them, just hearing them. Leave them and find a sound quite close to you, be aware of it without judgement, leave it and enter your own space.

Feel where your body touches the surface it
rests on.
Feel the spaces where the body doesn't touch.
Feel the clothes touching the body.
Feel your heart beating, sending blood
around your body to nourish you.
Feel the breath easily and lightly entering and
leaving your body.

*Using a meditation stool is excellent for the
posture, or use a comfortable straight-backed chair*

Cushions from Linen and Lace of Balmain

Breath is vital. Drawing in breath is the first thing we do when we are born and breathing out the last thing when we die. We can live for about four weeks without food, four days without water and four minutes without air and yet we have almost forgotten how to breathe. We take the air into the top few centimetres (inches) of our lungs and call it 'breathing' but our bodies are crying out for oxygen which is mainly denied.

Remember: shallow breathing creates tension; deep breathing releases tension. Watch the breath the next time you are afraid, anxious or angry. See how it is shallow and short. See what happens when the fear or anger passes—how you draw in a long, deep breath and relax.

Take your attention to your breath. Keep your shoulders loose and relaxed and forget about your chest.

Imagine that in your belly you have a balloon. A coloured balloon…red, orange, yellow…any colour you like. As you gently breathe in through your nose, the balloon inflates until it fills your belly space. As you breathe out through your mouth, the balloon slowly deflates until it's quite flat.

This method of breathing may be quite difficult at first but will become easier as you practise. When you are nervous, tense or angry, stop, drop your shoulders and take three or four deep 'belly breaths'. Your tension, anger or nervousness will begin to dissipate, leaving you in control once again.

Don't treat meditation as a chore; it's your special time so have fun with it. You may have five minutes or twenty minutes to spare—whatever you have, use and enjoy it.

A few meditations are outlined below. If one doesn't suit you, then move to another. Even the ones you enjoy may become stale and 'used' after a while—move to another.

These meditations direct your mind and give it something to do. If you make a conscious effort 'not to think' you will fail: within one or two seconds your mind will have found something to chatter about and will leap from one subject to another until, when you catch up with it, you find that the last thought is totally disconnected from the first.

Trying to 'force' the mind is an impossible task. To demonstrate this I say to meditation groups at the first session, 'Close your eyes; think of anything you like but don't think of a white horse'. Within seconds the whole group is laughing and one can almost 'hear the beat of the horses' hooves' as white horses canter through the meditation room!

If you give your attention to a specific subject it becomes a little easier to 'tame the monkey' but at first the mind will beat you and run around again. When this happens, don't lose patience, don't become angry—gently move the mind to one side and return to your meditation.

Use the relaxation methods and the breathing. At first, do only ten minutes of any of the meditations. Increase slowly. Feel the difference.

ONE

With each breath going out, say 'one' in your mind and see the word on the mind's screen.

As the breath goes out, say 'one'.
Breathe in gently—don't say anything.
Breathe out, saying and seeing 'one'. Feel that you are one with exercise.

BREATH WATCHING

Another simple meditation is 'breath watching', in which you breathe gently and easily in and through the nostrils.

Find the point where you feel the air entering your body.
It may be the opening of the nostrils, it may be the point where the nostrils join the back of the throat.
Feel the difference between the in-breath— and the out-breath.
If thoughts intrude, move them gently away and return to the watching.

MANTRAS

Mantras are incantations which have been used for centuries as a gate to meditation. Single-word mantras such as 'Aum' may be said out loud.

Two-syllable mantras are spoken in the mind and the heart. Be constantly aware of the significance and beauty of your mantra—watch that it doesn't become a word which you are repeating parrot fashion otherwise you might just as well be saying 'cellar door'.

The words 'love', 'peace', 'shanti' (peace), or any word or short phrase such as 'I am love' or 'peace and light' can be used as mantras. It doesn't actually matter what you say as long as it flows with the breathing and feels relaxing and positive.

SO-HAM

This ancient mantra means 'I am the One'. As you breathe in, say and see in your mind, 'so'. As you breathe out, say and see in your mind, 'ham'.

Sitting quietly, breathing easily, so…ham… so…ham…so…ham…

Over and over…Over and over—feel the words in your heart, don't just repeat them.

AUM (OM)

This word is the sound of the Universe. Try different notes and watch where in your body the sounds resonate and vibrate.

Say it slowly and out loud on the out-breath. AH-OH-OO-MMMMMMMMMMMM

POSITIVITY

SMILE

You can bring your inner smile to bloom when you wake, at times throughout the day, and any time you feel negative or are with negative people.

Imagine a smile curving along the bottom of your belly, following the natural curve which is there. Don't let the smile appear on your face. Now the smile begins to spread until the whole abdomen is filled with a big, curving smile. The smile fills your belly and chest. Now the smile blooms on your face and through your body.

THOUGHT STOPPING

When you are beset with seemingly insoluble problems which nibble and chew at your mind, give them your complete attention and ask a question: 'Is there anything I can do about the situation right now?' If the answer is 'Yes', then do it; even though it's difficult, do it.

If the answer is 'No, I can't do anything right now', try one of the following techniques.

➤ Distraction: When the worrying happens, tell your mind, 'I'm very sorry but I'm really busy right now. I promise faithfully that I will give you some attention in a little while, so please be patient.' In seconds, minutes or hours the problem will once again re-appear and you will repeat the sentence.

Keep doing this over and over again. When you finally say 'OK, now let's worry', you will probably find that the problem seems to have lost its significance or during the non-worrying time your subconscious has come up with a solution.

➤ 'STOP': This is a powerful technique which has been used successfully for a very long time.

When you are sick to death of this nagging in your brain, shout 'Stop'. If you are in a place where you can shout out loud, take a deep breath and go for it—as loudly as you can!

If it's not appropriate to shout out loud, take a deep breath and yell 'Stop' in your mind. You will be astonished at how loudly you can shout without making a sound. Worries are amazingly easily intimidated. They are not as powerful as they would have you believe. Every time the worries come, shout 'STOP'.

This has been only a brief introduction to meditation and relaxation methods but I hope that it has inspired you to want more. Meditation classes are helpful in the beginning. It's often much easier to meditate with other people.

Don't let anyone tell you that they will teach you the 'best' or the most 'correct' meditation—there is no such thing. There are as many ways to meditate as there are stars in the sky (nice meditation, counting stars!) and if you search, gently and with an open mind, you will find the perfect ones for you.

'TIME OUT'

By the time you reach this part of the book you might have cupboards bulging with moisture creams, scrubs, shampoos, massage oils and all the other good things which you have made! You will have read the chapter about relaxation and meditation and be ready to put it all into practice with some 'Time Out'.

'Time Out' is for everyone: women, men and children. Somehow the idea of taking time to cherish yourself seems to be confined to women (who rarely do it), but children enjoy pampering and are the best meditators, and men are slowly getting the idea that it's all right to take care of your body and soul.

Budget time in the same way as you budget money. Thirty minutes can be spent on: a facial steam, a pack or scrub, a manicure or pedicure, a walk or swim, a meditation. One hour can be spent on: a deep facial, a hair-conditioning treatment, a massage, a luxurious bath.

Half a day, or even one whole day a month can be spent as follows: Do a deal with the family: if each person has a 'Time Out' day each month or so, the rest of the family will relieve the family member of chores for this day. You will all feel more appreciative of each other and completely renewed after giving yourself this break. You might like to follow some or all of my suggestions or have ideas of your own.

➤ Sleep in as late as you want, have your favourite breakfast in bed, read a book, listen to some music, meditate—whatever.
➤ Prepare a facial steam and put it on to simmer. Prepare a hair rinse at the same time.
➤ Heat the bathroom if it's cold and collect everything you will need: body brush, shampoo, pre-shampoo treatment, after-shampoo conditioner, loofah, pumice, nail brush, bath salts or one of the bath oils or mixtures for the bath, soap, two big fluffy towels, a book, incense. Anything you need to feel relaxed and pampered.
➤ Apply a pre-shampoo treatment to your hair and put a shower cap on.

➤ Steam the face for five to ten minutes, splash with cool water.
➤ Make a mask such as Egg on Your Face.
➤ Begin to run the bath, adding anything you fancy from Chapter Four.
➤ Make a cup of your favourite drink, retire to the bathroom and shut the door. Ahhhhhhh!
➤ Body-brush from head to foot, shower if you like, climb into the bath.
➤ Spend as long as you like in the bath—sipping your drink, reading your book or just enjoying the luxury of doing nothing (this bit usually takes me about two hours and lots of topping up of water).
➤ When you are ready you can spread the mask on your face and then begin to pay some attention to your hands and feet. Scrub the nails, push the softened cuticles back very gently. Pumice any rough patches on soles or heels.
➤ Time to leave the bath and wash the face mask off in the shower with lukewarm water. Wash your hair with one of the herbal shampoos and rinses and finish with Herbal Hair Dressing.
➤ Wrap your head in a towel and dry your body. Massage some moisture lotion over your entire body and face and either put a dressing gown on or persuade someone to give you a massage.
➤ Time for another drink and maybe something to eat (my favourite is feta and avocado salad and my friend Nirala's home-made bread).
➤ Now set or brush your hair, file the nails on your hands and feet and massage in hand cream.
➤ This is the point where I dress, then take the dogs for a walk and call at the video store for a good movie. I must confess that this is also the time when I indulge my taste buds and buy some chocolate to go with the movie—an end to a perfect day!

This seems like a good point at which to end the main part of this book. I hope that you get a lot of pleasure from using it and that the contents helps to enhance your life. Treat it all as fun and above all—be happy!

Flowers by Lisa Milasas

Use home-made beauty products to pamper yourself when having 'Time Out'

GLOSSARY

ACACIA, GUM (*Acacia* sp.) Also called 'gum arabic'. Natural resin from the acacia (mainly *Acacia senegal*) which may be slowly dissolved in water to form a slightly acid, mucilaginous base for stabilising and thickening creams and lotions. The mucilage also forms the base for many sweets and pastilles where it is used as a thickener and soother. The gel is gentle and emollient to the skin. Acacia oxidises easily so care needs to be taken when including it in preparations to be used externally: either use a preservative or, alternatively, the oxydising enzyme can be inactivated by heating the mucilage to 100°C (212°F) for a short time. Acacia is often used in conjunction with tragacanth. Mild allergen.

ACID/ALKALINE Skin has an acid mantle with a pH which ranges between 5.5 and 6.2. This milk acidity protects the skin from invading bacteria. See also pH, below.

AGAR-AGAR This is a jelly preparation from seaweeds of various kinds. It can be used by vegetarians as a substitute for gelatine in internal and external preparations. Agar-agar doesn't set in quite the same way as gelatine: it has a more 'crisp' texture but has the advantage of having better setting qualities in hot weather.

ALCOHOLS Ethanol alcohol is a 95% proof alcohol and is used, at various dilutions, for making tinctures and astringents and for dissolving essential oils. In Australia and Britain it's not possible to buy this alcohol without a licence. Some pharmacists will sell small amounts if they know you as a responsible person. If you can't find a supply it's perfectly all right to use the highest proof alcohol available. Vodka, brandy, gin and other similar drinks are suitable. There is a Polish vodka which is 80% proof.

ALFALFA (*Medicago sativa*) Sprouts, seeds. We should eat this plant each week as the sprouts are rich in protein, calcium, trace elements, carotene and vitamins. Alfalfa contains protease (a protein digester) which acts as an exfoliant when included in creams and oils and facial steams. The ground seeds may also be mixed with other exfoliants such as pineapple for a mask. Mild allergen.

ALLERGEN A substance which creates an allergic reaction. There isn't a substance on this earth which won't cause an allergic reaction on someone but some substances are more likely than others to cause a problem. If you are allergy prone or have a sensitive skin it would be wise to 'patch test' doubtful substances before including them in products and using them on your body. To make a patch test, take a small amount of the herb you wish to test, make a paste with some ground herb and water, and place a blob inside your elbow. Cover with sticking plaster and leave for twenty-four hours. If there is no soreness, itching or redness you can safely go ahead and use the plant.

ALMOND (*Prunus dulcis*) Kernel. This is the sweet almond as opposed to the bitter almond. The kernel is ground and may be used as a gentle skin scrub or soaked in boiling water as a moisturising and softening skin milk (which is also delicious and nutritious as a drink).

ALOE (*Aloe vera*; *Aloe arborescens*) Leaves. Aloe vera is a plant of the aloe family with thick juicy leaves growing from a basal rosette. The leaves have spines down each side and the green surface is dotted with white 'spots'. This aloe can live happily in a pot in the kitchen where its juicy jelly is invaluable to soothe kitchen stove burns.

A. arborescens is a much taller plant whose leaves are longer, spinier and grow on a stem. I have found both types of aloe to be equally effective in creams and lotions where they soften, heal and soothe the skin. The leaf may be slit open to reveal a thick, clear jelly which can be applied direct to burns. To prepare aloe for use in creams and lotions, see Chapter One. Allergen.

ALTERATIVE   A loose term to describe the ability of a herb such as red clover (*Trifolium pratense*) to slowly change the condition of ill health to health.

ALUM   Double sulphate of aluminium and potassium. Colourless, transparent, odourless granular powder which is soluble in water. Alum is a powerful astringent and haemostatic.

People tend to shy like frightened horses at the mention of aluminium and while I would agree that it's not good to ingest too much aluminium (there is now concern that high intakes of aluminium may increase permeability of the brain—allowing undesirable substances to penetrate—and may be a contributor to Alzheimer's disease), many authorities claim that ingested aluminium is not absorbed into the blood stream but passes through the intestines and is excreted.There is no evidence to show that alum is absorbed when applied externally against perspiration or to stop bleeding. Alum precipitates and binds with proteins which are excreted in sweat and which decompose very rapidly unless this action takes place. Alum should be used as a 2% solution (2g in 100ml/3^{1}/$_{3}$fl oz water) and provided it is not increased it is considered safe to use. Alum hardens skin and so is a useful addition to foot preparations where it prevents blistering.

ANGELICA (*Angelica archangelica*)   Leaves, seeds, root. A large handsome biannual herb which is a stimulant and a useful addition to skin tonics.

ANISE (*Pimpinella anisum*)   Seeds. An annual herb with delicious liquorice-scented and liquorice-flavoured seeds. Use the crushed seeds in facial steams, where it is an aid in the treatment of acne, and as an infusion for a rinse to cleanse the scalp.

ANTIFUNGAL   A substance which inhibits the growth of fungus. Benzoin (*Styrax benzoin*) is an example.

ANTISEPTIC   An agent which inhibits bacteria growth on living tissue and prevents sepsis. Calendula (*Calendula officinalis*) is a powerful antiseptic.

APPLE (*Pyrus malus*)   Flesh. The pulp makes a mild, naturally acid pack for sensitive skin particularly if mixed with a little honey. Diluted apple cider vinegar is a useful hair rinse and skin tonic—its mild acidity has astringent and antibacterial actions.

APRICOT (*Prunus armeniaca*)   Flesh. Acne and oily skin sufferers may benefit from using a mask of crushed apricots (fresh or reconstituted dried). The flesh is naturally acidic and is full of vitamin A. Apricot oil is a wonderfully rich emollient to include in moisturising creams and lotions.

AROMATHERAPY   A system which uses volatile oils (also called 'essential oils') to treat physical and mental complaints by massage or inhalation. For more information, see Chapter Six.

AROMATIC   A plant or medicine which has an agreeable smell/taste. Aromatic herbs are often used to disguise an unpleasant taste in herbal compounds. Liquorice (*Glycyrrhiza glabra*) is one of the most popular aromatics.

ARROWROOT (*Maranta arundinacea, canna edulis*)   Rhizomes. The rhizomes from these plants are pounded, washed and strained to produce a powdered starch called arrowroot. This powder makes an excellent soothing body powder and deodorant. With other constituents it can be made into a treatment for pimples (see Chapter Two).

In cooking it is used as for cornflour but seems to be a safer thickener to use, as the plant is not subject to insecticidal spraying.

ASCORBIC ACID   Another name for vitamin C. Useful to create an acid pH in preparations and as an antioxidant for oily preparations. Mix 2 teaspoons ascorbic acid powder with 2 teaspoons water (or as much as is needed to dissolve the powder). Add, a drop at a time, to finished creams to adjust the pH to as near 5.0 as possible.

ASTRINGENT   An agent which has the power to contract tissues. Plantains (*Plantago major, P. lanceolata*) are examples of astringent herbs.

BANANA   Flesh. The mashed fruit makes a soothing, nourishing face mask. Don't waste the peels: pack around the base of your rose trees, cover with a little soil and the rose bush will reward you with bigger, more beautiful blooms.

BASIL (*Ocymum basilicum*) Leaves. A deliciously aromatic annual herb with drawing properties. Basil is useful (pounded) for drawing out the poison and easing the pain of bee or ant stings. The pulp will also bring pimples to a head. It is best used fresh.

Taken internally as an infusion, basil eases stomach cramps and vomiting, increases appetite and, if in food, helps to prevent indigestion.

Basil oil is combined with lavender and rosemary oils to make a sweet-smelling, tonic hair oil.

BARLEY Used in cooking, barley is nutritious, emollient and very easy to digest. Barley water is good for people with bladder problems as it soothes and cleanses. If I had a fever as a child I would be given lots of lemon barley water to drink. The water used from boiled barley is a soothing additive to a bath. Use for sunburn, eczema, itchy skin and dry skin.

BEANS Green beans contain a principle which seems to have a curative effect on psoriasis, eczema, dandruff and other skin diseases. Chop the beans and use them to make an infusion. Drink a cupful three times a day. Use the same infusion as a skin and scalp wash.

BEETROOT Flesh or root. A highly nutritious vegetable, particularly if grated and eaten raw. The juice squeezed from finely grated beetroot and reduced by simmering in a double boiler can be incorporated in lip salves and moisture creams to give a rosy glow to lips and cheeks.

BEESWAX A wax, secreted by bees, which forms the cell walls of the honeycomb. Beeswax is an ideal wax to use in ointments and creams. When combined with borax it makes an emulsifying wax.

It's possible to buy bleached white beeswax from pharmacies in pieces or in small buttons. I understand that it becomes hypoallergenic when treated in this way. I like to use the natural wax.

If you buy your wax direct from an apiarist it is likely to contain contaminants—bees' legs and wings, bits of plant matter and so on. To prepare the wax for use, see Chapter One. Mild allergen.

BENZOIN (*Styrax benzoin*) Resin which is collected from incisions made in the bark of the tree and allowed to harden. The hard lumps of resin are then collected. They may be powdered and used as a fixative in potpourris (add 10–30% by weight; that is, 10–30g ($^1/_3$–1oz) benzoin to 100g ($3^1/_3$oz) dried plant material); added to soap for the antiseptic, antibacterial and antifungal properties; made into a tincture and used as a preservative in creams, ointments etc. The tincture can be used for eczema, blackheads, boils, pimples and itching.

Note: If you buy the tincture from a pharmacy be sure that you buy only Simple Tincture of Benzoin. Compound tincture of benzoin (also known as Friar's Balsam) has other additives which may be harmful if used incorrectly.

It seems to be increasingly difficult to buy the simple tincture but gum benzoin is more readily available through health food stores or herb wholesalers making it simple to make a tincture.

BERGAMOT (*Monarda didyma*) Leaves and flowers. Also known as 'bee balm' or 'Oswego tea'. Bergamot is a perennial, shade-loving herb whose perfumed leaves and bright red flowers are used in teas, potpourris, sachets, facial steams and masks. The oil (not to be confused with *Citrus bergamia*—see below) is used to perfume cosmetics. The infusion made from bergamot is the famous 'Oswego tea' drunk by North American Indians and by Americans during the time of the tea embargo. The tea is delicious and eases nausea, vomiting and flatulence.

BERGAMOT OIL An essential oil extract from the rind of the tree *Citrus bergamia*. Mild allergen.

BICARBONATE OF SODA (SODIUM BICARBONATE) Otherwise known as baking soda. It eases pain quickly if made into a paste with vinegar and applied to stings or ant bites. Mixed with salt an makes a great tooth cleaner (see Chapter Two).

BORAGE (*Borago officinalis*) Leaves, flowers. An annual plant with beautiful blue flowers. Borage is a 'cooling' herb and an infusion is useful as a drink when there is fever present and also as a revitaliser during convalescence. An infusion of the flowers and leaves may be used as a soothing cold compress to ease a headache or strained as an eye lotion. Allergen.

Note: The lotion must be strained through coffee filter paper, as the leaves are covered in hairs which could be dangerous.

BORAX (SODIUM TETRABORATE)   A mineral collected from the shores of alkaline lakes. Borax is mildly alkaline and softening and may be used effectively in many cosmetic products. Combined with beeswax it will make a stable emulsion. Don't use internally, on broken skin, or for babies.

BRAN   The husk of grains such as oats, barley and wheat. Bran may be used as a substitute for, or mixed with, oats as a water softener in recipes for bath bags. It is also a useful ingredient in facial scrubs. Bran is a valuable addition to our food intake as it acts as a natural laxative.

BREWER'S YEAST   A by-product of beer and ale brewing. Brewer's yeast is a valuable food additive as it's a rich source of B vitamins, protein, chromium and selenium. Mixed with yoghurt it makes an excellent mask for oily skins. It is too stimulating to be used on sensitive or very dry skins.

BRUISE   A method used to help a plant to release its properties into liquids, such as oils, vinegars, and water. The seed, root or leaf is tapped firmly with a hard object such as a pestle using enough pressure to break the outer covering but not to mash or crush completely.

BURDOCK (*Arctium lappa*)   Mainly root. Is antibacterial and fungicidal. A biennial herb with a large root. An infusion of dried, ground root is used in facial steams, baths, compresses, poultices and infusions. Burdock is a fine 'blood cleanser' so may be used (as a tincture or decoction) internally as well as externally to gain the full effect from its properties. A decoction of grated root is particularly useful as a wash against fungal diseases of the skin eg athlete's foot.

CALENDULA (*Calendula officinalis*)   Mainly petals. This is one of my favourites. Sunny, friendly and obliging—once you have planted them they will self-seed and pop up all over the garden forever. They will appear in the vegetable garden and in the herb beds. In ointments, creams, lotions and tinctures I only use the petals for their golden yellow colour and softening, antiseptic action.

CARROTS   Flesh. Carrots contain lots of betacarotene. I make a rich golden yellow oil from carrots, comfrey and calendula petals to use in dry/normal skin moisturisers. A cleansing mask can be made from cooked mashed carrots.

CASTILE SOAP   A soap made from olive oil and other ingredients. Many years ago soap would need to contain 40–50% olive oil in order to be recognised as 'Castile Soap'. These days the oil content need be no more than 20%. Hard castile soap with a high proportion of olive oil is sometimes difficult to buy but there are now some lovely liquid castile soaps on the market which are very pleasant. You can make castile soap using one of the recipes in Chapter Five.

CHAMOMILE (*Matricaria chamomilla*)   Common name: German chamomile; (*Anthemis nobilis*) Common name: Roman chamomile.   Mainly flowers. I would imagine that the chamomiles are probably among the best known herbs. German chamomile is an annual plant. This is the chamomile used internally as an infusion as Roman chamomile is very bitter. The medicinal benefits to be obtained are so many that I would refer my book *Herbcraft* for the list.

The blue oil 'azulene' is distilled from *Matricaria chamomilla*. An infusion of either of the chamomiles applied as a compress will soothe, cleanse and reduce puffiness of the skin (particularly of the face). If carefully strained, the infusion may be used as a compress for sore, puffy and tired eyes.

Flowers from the chamomiles contain a non-volatile oil called 'apigenin' which gives light hair a lighter tone and is therefore useful in shampoos and rinses for restoring colour to fair hair. Mild allergen.

CHICKWEED (*Stellaria media*)   Whole herb. An annual herb with plenty of little white, star-shaped flowers, considered by many to be a 'weed' as it grows so profusely in the spring. Don't despise this plant, as it comes at the time of year when we need infusions of the whole herb as a 'spring tonic'.

I once treated a six-month-old baby who had

suffered from severe eczema since birth. He was given a weak infusion of chickweed tea to drink, litres of triple strength infusion (see Chapter One) were poured into his bath and he was 'basted' with the water! After the bath, the worst areas were treated with chickweed ointment. As he was a breastfed baby his mother also drank infusions of the herb. Within two weeks the eczema had completely disappeared.

CHLOROCRESOL   See PRESERVATIVES.

CITRIC ACID   As the name suggests, this is an acid extracted from citrus fruits. It is useful for creating an acid pH in home-made skin and hair preparations and for inhibiting oxidisation in oily creams and ointments. See also ASCORBIC ACID.

CLARY SAGE (*Salvia sclarea*)   Leaves. A biennial plant of the sage family with large rough grey-green leaves. The oil is used as a fixative and a 'moderator' in perfumes and is therefore an ingredient of many perfumed products. The dried leaves will act as a fixative in potpourris. The seeds may be used to make an eye lotion, and an infusion of the dried leaves (which have an astringent effect) may be used for baths or toners.

COCOA BUTTER (*Theobroma cacao*)   Big rollers are used to press this delicious smelling fat from the cocoa bean of the cacao. The fat has a very low melting point and even though it looks similar to beeswax, unlike beeswax it liquefies much more easily on the skin. Cocoa butter is a superb rich emollient for dry skin, pregnant tummies and breasts. Use alone or in creams and lotions to soften and protect skin particularly in the areas where the skin is thinnest—around the eyes, lips and throat. (For these preparations, see Chapter Two.) Mild allergen.

COLTSFOOT (*Tussilago farfara*)   Leaves. A perennial herb with hoof-shaped leaves (hence the name) which is emollient and astringent. Externally it is used as a wash to treat thread veins, inflammations and swellings. A single strength infusion strained through coffee filter paper can be used as an eye wash for sore and tired eyes. Tea may be taken as anti-inflammatory andto heal skin problems.

COMFREY (*Symphytum officinale*)   Leaves in summer, root in winter. A perennial herb with hairy, coarse leaves. The main active ingredient is allantoin. Comfrey has attracted the attention of the Commonwealth Department of Health and in 1984 was listed as a Schedule 1 poison. This means that there is a ban on its internal use unless prescribed by persons licensed to sell Schedule 1 poisons. The ban applies to the dried plant only, which is illogical as there is a far higher level of alkaloids present in the fresh plant. There are more potentially hazardous substances present in foods which are freely available on the grocer's shelves: nitrates (used in cured meats); artificial colours and flavours; monosodium glutamate; sulphur (used to prevent dried foods from discolouring) and many more.

Allantoin, the active constituent of comfrey, is used in many reputable pharmaceuticals! As an external remedy, comfrey stands alone in the treatment of cuts and bruises. Its emollient and healing properties are valuable in creams, lotions, ointments, shampoos and baths. Mild allergen.

COMPRESS   A method of applying cold, stimulation, moisture or the healing properties of various agents to areas of the body. A compress is made by soaking a cloth in cold liquid. If the compress is to be used on the face, never apply it too hot or too cold to areas where it could 'break' tiny capillaries.

CORNMEAL   Cornmeal is dried ground corn which can be used in facial masks and body scrubs, and as a mild exfollient in soap and facial scrubs. Rubbed into hair it will absorb the grease and is easier to brush out than many other dry shampoos.

CUCUMBER (*Cucumis sativa*)   This is one of the very best vegetables (internally and externally) for skin care as it's full of minerals and vitamins necessary for the health of skin, nails and hair. The juice is astringent, soothing, cooling and softening. The main astringency is in the flesh, so when using externally, if you have oily skin, peel the cucumber; if your skin is dry or normal, leave the skin on to reduce the astringency. The juice can be strained and used in lotions, tonics, creams and sunburn-soothers. Whole slices laid on the closed eyes take the sting and burn out of tired strained eyes and help to reduce under-eye puffiness.

DAIRY PRODUCTS   Milk, cream, buttermilk, dried skim milk powder, butter and yoghurt all have many uses in skin care for softening, moisturising, refining, smoothing and soothing.

DANDELION (*Taraxacum officinale*)   Leaf and root. Dandelion coffee drunk three times a day would do more for the appearance than most cosmetics. Dandelion, the 'liver' herb, promotes the formation of bile and has a diuretic action on the kidneys. These properties help to cleanse our bodies of the toxins which can be responsible for giving us lacklustre eyes and sallow skin. The leaves are rich in vitamins A and C and are useful in facial steams, packs and washes for treatment of skin complaints.

DECOCTION   Roots, barks and seeds usually need to be simmered to extract their properties. The resulting liquid is called a decoction. For more information, see Chapter One.

DEMULCENT   An agent which soothes and lubricates internally. An example is mallow (*Althoea* sp.).

DIAPHORETIC   An agent which promotes perspiration. An example is yarrow (*Achillea millefolium*).

DIGESTIVE   An agent which helps digestion. An example is fennel (*Foeniculum vulgare*).

DISINFECTANT   A substance which destroys bacteria and so helps to prevent disease.

DIURETIC   An agent such as dandelion (*Taraxacum officinale*) which causes a freer flow of urine.

DOCK (*Rumex* sp.)   Root. The roots of all the dock family are astringent and can be made into mouthwashes to strengthen gums and teeth. The dried, ground root can be used as a toothpowder.

DOUCHE   The introduction of fluid into the body, usually the vagina, using a special douche bag which contains infusions or decoctions to help in the healing of various vaginal infections.

EGGS   Probably as old a beauty aid as milk and butter. The yolk is rich and nourishing for dry skins while the white is especially useful for oily skins (it might prove too drying for sensitive, dry skin). Whipped white of egg will temporarily tighten puffy skin—very useful if you look a wreck and need a quick facelift! Whole eggs may be used in face packs and as a conditioner for hair (don't use very hot water to rinse or you'll end up with strands of cooked egg on your head!).

ELDER (*Sambucus canadensis, S. nigra*)   Flowers, fruit and leaves. The elder tree has huge clusters of aromatic, creamy white flowers which are used internally as a diaphoretic tea to ease the miseries of colds and flu. Externally, the flowers are used as refreshing and cleansing skin washes; as a lotion to fade freckles; as a gentle skin tonic; as an eyewash; and are added to baths to ease itchy or sunburnt skin. Don't forget to ask permission from the Elder Mother before taking any part of her tree or she might vent her wrath on your household!

EMOLLIENT   An agent used to soothe external inflammation or dryness. Comfrey (*Symphytum officinale*) has emollient properties.

EMULSIFYING WAX   An emulsifier is an agent which blends oils and water together as an homogenous mixture. There are many types of emulsifying agents but the two which I have found to be the most stable are cetomacrogol emulsifying wax and stearic acid. The latter makes a wonderful, light vanishing cream but needs the addition of triethanolamine (see later). There are simple emulsifying agents such as beeswax, lecithin and borax with which you might like to experiment but they don't have the same stability as cetamacrogol and stearic acid.

ENFLEURAGE   A method of extracting essential oil from petals of flowers, in particular, jasmine and tuberose. See Chapter Six.

EPSOM SALTS (MAGNESIUM SULPHATE)   A mineral salt originally obtained from the springs at Epsom in Surrey. Epsom salts is an excellent additive to baths, where it eases tired bodies and aching muscles, and to foot baths for those times when 'your feet are killing you'. Made into a poultice it draws boils and pimples to a head.

ESSENCE   A mixture of essential oil and alcohol; for the purpose of this book an essence is a mixture of 15ml (½fl oz) oil with 1 cup (250ml/8fl oz) high proof vodka. This is a 6% solution.

Examples of essences which could be used in the kitchen would be peppermint and vanilla essence. Essences have many uses such as in perfumes, deodorants, and house sprays.

ESSENTIAL FATTY ACIDS   Fatty acids which cannot be produced by the body but must be supplied in the diet. See also HYDROGENATION.

EUCALYPTS (*Eucalyptus globulus* and sp.)   Leaves. The leaves of many of the common eucalypts may be crushed and used in boiling water as an inhalation to clear the nasal passages or used in the bath mixtures for their antiseptic properties. I like to use the leaves and the essential oil when I make the base oil for healing ointments. For uses of the essential oil, see Chapter Six.

EXFOLIANT   An agent used to peel dead cells gently from the surface of the skin.

FENNEL (*Foeniculum vulgare*)   Mainly seeds. Fennel grows like a weed in Australia, particularly along railway embankments. The seeds lessen the pangs of hunger and I'm told that Italian railway workers would chew the seeds to help them through the hours until 'smoko'. Fennel seeds are a pleasant way to ensure well-digested food. Even the most humble cafe in India has little dishes of the seeds on the tables for patrons to nibble after their meal and we always had these digestives on the tables at our restaurant, The Prancing Pony. Fennel tea is said to increase the milk supply of nursing mothers. Externally, fennel seeds or leaves are added to facial steams and eye washes. The delicious aroma of the crushed seeds makes it a nice addition to soaps and perfumes.

FIXATIVE   Usually a 'base note' essential oil used to fix the more fleeting perfumes of top and middle notes. Clove and patchouli are examples.

FIXED OILS   Natural, usually non-volatile oils, occurring in the seeds, kernels, beans, etc. of plants and extracted by presses, chemicals or heat. Fixed oils are fats which are liquid at room temperature. (Not to be confused with the 'aromatic' or essential oils; for these oils, see Chapter Six.) There is considerable dispute regarding the benefits of 'cold-pressed' versus chemically extracted oils. I am assured by a very reputable pharmaceutical chemist that the solvent used to dissolve oils from the base seed or fruit is evaporated off at a low temperature and that no trace remains in the oil at the end of the process; also that the nutritional content remains the same. He added further that on analysis it is impossible to differentiate between the oils treated chemically or by cold pressing.

In her book, *Health on your Plate*, Janette Pleshette presents a totally different perspective. She says that the oil-bearing materials go through fifteen separate processes involving chemical solvents, caustic soda and deodorants which remove lecithin, vitamin E and minerals. She goes on to state that; 'The heat used in refining oils can reach about 235°C (about 455°F). The oils are often held at this high level for several hours and it is this prolonged heat which is damaging.' She also states: 'We have seen that refining oils destroys most of their nutrients…'

Cold-pressed oils are perceived by many as being preferable because there has been no chemical or heat applied in the extraction process. The term 'cold-pressed' is a misnomer as the pressure used in the press causes the heat to rise to 120°C (250°F); this is, however, far less than the refining process. (If you are interesting in finding out more, I urge you to read Janette Pleshette's book —I list it in the Book List at the back of this book.)

The ultimate choice of oils must be yours, dictated by your preferences and (up to a point) your purse.

Oils are classified as:

(a) Non-drying   Non-drying oils contain mainly oleic acid glycerides, very little linoleic or linolenic acids. They remain liquid at normal temperatures and do not form a film when exposed to oxygen. These are the oils which are most suitable for dry and normal skins and are the main ones to use in massage oils.

(b) Semi-drying   These oils contain more linoleic and linolenic acids, dry slowly to a soft film when exposed to oxygen and are suitable for dry to normal skins. These oils should only be used in small quantities in massage oils.

(c) Drying   Drying oils are high in linoleic and linolenic acids, low in oleic acids and dry quite quickly to a tough, elastic film when exposed to oxygen. These oils are often added to paints to shorten the drying time. Drying oils are not advised for inclusion in massage oils as they would form a film on the skin, but may be included in creams and lotions as the combination of ingredients during emulsification alters the character of the oil.

It's wise to keep oils in the refrigerator to help to delay oxidisation/rancidity for as long as possible.

ALMOND OIL, BITTER   The delicious scent of this oil, expressed from the kernel of the bitter almond (*Prunis amygdalus*), makes it a popular addition to perfumes and soaps. The unprocessed oil contains prussic acid which by law must be removed before the oil is offered for sale.

ALMOND OIL, SWEET   A fine, emollient, non-drying oil expressed from the kernel of the sweet almond (*Prunis communis dulcis*). An excellent oil to use in creams, lotions and massage oils formulated for dry, normal and combination skins.

APRICOT KERNEL OIL   A pale yellow oil obtained from the kernel of the apricot seed. Contains minerals and vitamins. A light, non-drying/semi-drying oil which is suitable for all skins especially mature, sensitive and dry.

AVOCADO OIL   A beautiful thick, green semi-drying oil. According to Mrs Carl F. Leyel in her book *Herbal Delights*, 'Avocado Pear oil…used as a cosmetic, has greater powers of penetration than any other vegetable oil…it conveys vitamins and nourishment to the glands that lie beneath the skin.' The oil contains vitamins A, D, E and K, is rich, nourishing and is invaluable in moisture creams and lotions, particularly for sensitive and sunburnt skins. The vitamin E content helps to preserve other oils in blends. Because of its thick consistency it's best to use no more than 5–10% in massage and face oils.

CANOLA OIL   Canola seed is modified rape seed. Rape seed oil has been under a cloud due to the presence of eructic acid which, when eaten in large quantities showed a fat accumulation in the heart muscle of animals. Canola was bred to be genetically low in eructic acid. This process was carried out in Canada hence the first three letters of the name.

Canola is a non-drying oil which is excellent in massage oils and in creams and lotions for dry and normal skins. It is also good for cooking as it is light and has little flavour of its own. If you like the taste of butter but don't want to eat so much saturated fat you could beat some canola oil into softened butter. This gives a spreadable consistency, less saturated fat and the benefits of monounsaturated fat. Unfortunately it still has the same number of kilojoules (calories)!

CASTOR OIL   A rich non-drying oil pressed from the seeds of the castor oil plant (*Ricinis communis*). (The seeds themselves are very poisonous.) It is an invaluable oil for use in hair conditioners, and in hot packs on sore muscles or to draw splinters which are deeply embedded in the flesh. It is richly emollient if included in small quantities in night creams and soaps. Note: Not recommended for internal use—can cause severe 'griping' pains.

COCONUT OIL   Coconut oil is a semi-solid saturated fat extracted from the white meat of the coconut. It is a wonderful lubricant and moisturiser for delicate eye and throat areas. If used very discreetly it conditions and gives a glossy shine to hair. It's sometimes possible to buy saponified coconut oil to make shampoos and bath foams. If refrigerated it remains solid but liquefies easily when at room temperature.

COPHA   An Australian product made entirely from hydrogenated coconut oil. This white waxy solid is much cheaper than coconut oil and may be used in creams, ointments and soaps.

CORN OIL   A good cosmetic oil, but Jeanne Rose in *The Herbal Body Book* comments 'I cannot recommend its use since a large percentage of the pesticides and fungicides that are employed in this country (the US) are used on corn'. I haven't been able to establish if the situation is the same in other countries so it becomes a case of 'let the buyer beware'. The other disadvantage of corn oil is it goes rancid more quickly than most other oils.

EVENING PRIMROSE OIL   Expressed from the seeds of evening primrose (*Oenothera biennis*), a tall, weedy herb with yellow flowers. The oil taken internally has many therapeutic uses such as for premenstrual syndrome, menopausal problems, heart disease, skin conditions and multiple sclerosis. It is a soothing, healing oil when added to creams and blends to help heal eczema, psoriasis and other inflammatory skin conditions. Use 10% in massage oils or blends.

GRAPESEED OIL   As the name suggests, this oil is pressed from grape seeds. It's a fine, semi-drying, polyunsaturated oil which makes it suitable for most skins except the very oily. It is a very good basic carrier oil as it is light, clear and has no smell. Add 5–10% wheat germ oil to help prevent rancidity.

HAZELNUT OIL   A fine yellow oil pressed from the kernel of the hazelnut. This oil contains vitamins, minerals and protein and is good for all skins. If you are feeling reckless and want to make a superlative cream or oil, 100% hazelnut oil may be used but as this oil is becoming increasingly difficult to buy you may want to use it more sparingly.

JOJOBA OIL   A yellow waxy oil pressed from the bean of the desert plant *Simmondsia chinensis*. It contains a waxy substance, similar to collagen, which gives skin a silky smooth feel. Useful for acne, eczema, hair conditioner, inflamed skin and psoriasis. Penetrates deeply. Use 10% in blends.

MINERAL/PARAFFIN OIL (BABY OIL)   Not much good for anyone and certainly not for babies! It is used extensively by cosmetic companies in cleansers, moisture creams and lotions because it's cheap, hypoallergenic and is completely inert which gives it indefinite shelf life. If used alone it remains on the surface of the skin but once incorporated in an emulsion it is absorbed into the skin in the same way as other oils. The only advantage that this oil has for home users is it doesn't go rancid.

Many books on natural cosmetics state that mineral oil leaches the vitamins from the skin— this is not strictly accurate. All oils used both internally and externally will collect fat soluble vitamins (A, D, E, K) as they travel through the body, but natural oils are then absorbed through the intestines, hence the vitamins aren't lost. Mineral oil isn't absorbed into the intestinal wall and the oil is excreted, along with the vitamins.

OLIVE OIL   A rich non-drying oil expressed from ripe olives. It is one of my favourites and I use cold-pressed Extra Virgin (how on earth can you have 'extra' virgin—you either are or you aren't!) which is from the first pressing and is very green and aromatic. Some people don't like the smell, they could try the lighter olive oils from later pressings.

Olive oil is too rich for oily skins but is excellent for massage oils, creams, soaps and lotions for dry and normal skins. A lovely oil to use on baby skin. This oil contains 80% oleic acid (described later).

PALM OIL   A non-drying oil expressed from the kernel of the fruit of the palm tree. Palm oil has similar properties to coconut oil. It is used commercially in the manufacture of soap.

PEACH KERNEL OIL   Same as apricot kernel oil.

PEANUT OIL (ARACHIS OIL)   A pale yellow non-drying oil with a faint, pleasant nutty odour and bland nutty taste. It contains protein, vitamins and minerals. It is good for dry and normal skins and may be used in the same way as olive oil.

SAFFLOWER OIL   A semi-drying, polyunsaturated oil obtained from the seed of the safflower. Contains protein, vitamins and minerals. This oil is an excellent 'all-rounder', good for balancing other oils in preparations and may be used, mixed with other oils, in massage oils, soaps, moisture creams and lotions and bath oils. Safflower oil needs refrigeration to delay oxidisation.

SESAME OIL   A semi-drying oil expressed from ripe sesame seeds. Contains protein, vitamins, minerals, lecithin. It is useful in all moisturising creams and lotions. Sesame oil absorbs ultraviolet rays so it may be used in suntanning preparations.

SOY OIL   An unsaturated drying oil expressed from the soya bean. Contains protein, vitamins and minerals. A little soy oil can be used in cleansing creams, moisturisers, massage and bath oils.

SUNFLOWER OIL   This is a semi-drying oil which may be used (even by those with oily skin) on throats and around the eyes where there are few oil glands and very thin skin.

VEGETABLE OIL   This is a broad term to cover a mixture of oils. They're chosen for their cost or availability at the time. The problems connected with using vegetable oil in preparations is there may be a mixture of canola, sunflower, safflower, soy or others—all good but with different properties, as discussed in FIXED OILS.

WHEAT GERM OIL   This is a richly nourishing fine, healing oil. The vitamin E content makes it useful for most skins, especially dry, prematurely aged skin or for eczema or psoriasis etc. Good in 'anti-stretch mark' blends. Helps to preserve other oils. Ten per cent is a valuable addition to creams, lotions, massage oils and soaps.

FLAX (*Linum usitatissimum*)   Seeds. Otherwise known as 'linseed'. The seeds are emollient and healing. If a speck of grit or other irritant is on the eyeball it can be painlessly, safely and easily removed by slipping a silky flax seed under the bottom eyelid. The seed swells to form a jelly and picks up the grit. The jelly then slides to the corner of the eye where it is easily removed. Obviously you would only use this method with a simple problem; if metal or similar has penetrated the eyeball you should get professional help immediately.

FOMENTATION   The use of hot wet cloths to ease pain and reduce inflammation. A fomentation is made by soaking a cloth in hot liquid. If the fomentation is to be used on the face—never apply too hot to areas where it could 'break' the tiny capillaries.

FULLER'S EARTH   This is a fine, naturally occurring mineral clay which ranges in colour from white to grey-green. It may be used as an oil-absorbing, cleansing and thickening agent in soaps, packs and masks (mainly for oily skins). The absorbent property makes it a useful dry shampoo for oily hair or footpowder for sweaty feet! The clay was used in the textile industry to remove grease (to 'full') from woollen fabric—hence the name.

GARLIC (*Allium sativum*)   Bulb. Probably the most used herb. We use garlic every day in one way or another: cooking; dog food (to deter fleas and pinworms); garden sprays; to soothe earache (see my book *Herbcraft*); and on pimples or sores.

GELATINE   A setting agent obtained from animal bones, hoofs and skin. It is rich in protein. Use it in cleansing gels, hair-setting lotions and conditioners as a thickener and protein additive. Vegetarians will find Agar-agar a good substitute.

GERANIUM (*Pelargonium* sp.)   Mainly leaves. There are so many varieties of geranium that entire books have been devoted to these plants. The essential oils extracted from these plants are used widely in perfumery, soap making and potpourris. A decoction of the root of the wild geranium *Geranium maculatum* is an excellent astringent and is used as a deodorant, styptic, vaginal douche, and tonic for oily skins. The leaves and flowers of other varieties are used for potpourris, facial steams, baths, masks and, in fact, are used anywhere that you find that you can employ the wonderful perfumes of the geraniums.

GLYCERINE   Glycerine is a natural substance present in animal and vegetable fats. It is usually obtained as a by-product of soap making. It is syrupy in consistency, colourless, odourless, sticky and sweet. If used in small proportions in lotions, creams and toners it acts as an antibacterial, softener, lubricant and humectant (holding moisture to the skin). If more than 20% is used in any recipe it will have the opposite effect and draw water from the skin. Adding a little glycerine to colognes gives a softness to an after-shower splash.

GRAPES (*Vitis vinifera*)   Fruit. The grape is an acidic fruit which makes it ideal for using on our naturally acidic skin. The skin relies on this acidity to repel bacteria. Most soaps are alkaline and while the skin is adept at restoring the acid mantle (using within half an hour) it's good to use slightly acid preparations as much as possible so that the skin is not exposed to risk. The mashed pulp of seedless grapes (unless you don't mind seeding them) mixed with other ingredients or used alone, makes a soothing, cooling, nourishing mask.

HENNA (*Lawsonia inermis*)   Leaves. The powdered dried leaves are used for the well-known hair dye. Less well known is the fact that the flowers (difficult to get in Australia) are sweetly perfumed and are lovely in sachets. The essence from the flower is also used in massage oils and perfumes.

HERBAL TEA BAGS   If you haven't much time to spare, a herbal tea bag makes a good 'quickie' bath bag. The tea made from the bag may also be used to mix face packs, creams and lotions—in fact anywhere that a herbal infusion is needed. Used chamomile tea bags make good eye compresses.

HOMEOPATHY   A system of healing which uses minute doses of herbs, minerals and other substances which, in large doses, would cause similar symptoms to those being suffered by the patient. Hippocrates first formed the concept that 'like cures like'. The idea was made popular in the Western world by Samuel Hahnemann (1755–1843).

HONEY   What a versatile and wonderful substance! It lends its soothing properties whether taken internally or used on the skin. A spoonful of honey in a cup of chamomile tea will ensure a good night's sleep—the honey helps the body to retain fluid so a trip to the toilet in the night is avoided. A tablespoon of honey and the same of cider vinegar in a glass of water ensures good bowel action. Externally honey acts as a moisturiser, skin softener and healer. Add a little to creams, soaps, masks and lotions or apply to spots and blemishes.

HOPS (*Humulus lupulus*)   Flowers. The dried flower of the female hop plant is a sedative. Added to other herbs it makes a soothing 'sleep' pillow. The scent of the flower when used alone is a little sickly so try adding lavender and lemon verbena.

HORSERADISH (*Armoracia lapanthifolia*)   Root. The root of the plant is used in the kitchen to make horseradish cream or sauce. The pungent root can be infused into a base oil to make a powerful massage oil for aching muscles. Mild allergic.

HORSETAIL (*Equisetum arvense*)   Stems. Horsetails are in a botanical class of their own. They are relics of the Carboniferous period and the hollow-jointed stems with no leaves look prehistoric. These plants are so rich in silica that country folk used to clean their saucepans with crumpled bunches of the herb. If you have problem nails and hair, infusions of this herb can supply the silica which you probably lack. The silica also strengthens connective tissue such as muscles and ligaments.

HUMECTANT   A substance which has the capacity for attracting and holding moisture in the skin. Glycerine and honey are humectants.

HYDROGENATION   A process using hydrogen by which liquid oils are converted into solid fats such as margarine. Hydrogenation produces abnormal EFA (essential fatty acids)—these are mirror images of normal EFA. The body accepts these and attempts to use them but by the time it finds that the atoms of the molecules are arranged in the wrong 'shape', the process has gone too far to abandon them and begin with normal EFA; the normal EFA are blocked out. The result of this is the use of hydrogenated products deprive the body of EFA. According to the British medical journal *The Lancet*, 'The hydrogenation plants of our modern food industry may turn out to have contributed to the causation of major disease'.

HYPERPIGMENTATION   Excessive skin pigmentation caused by overexposure to sun or use of plants which cause photosensitivity.

INFUSION   The simplest and most widely used herbal preparation, in which boiling water is poured over herbs to make a tea. See Chapter One.

INHALATION   A method of clearing mucus and healing infection in the sinuses and respiratory system by breathing in aromatic steam made by adding herbs, essential oils etc. to boiling water.

IRISH MOSS (*Chondrus crispus*)   Not a moss but a seaweed, also called 'carrageenan'. The plant is emollient, soothing and very good for ageing skins. It acts as an emulsion stabiliser and thickener in creams and lotions.

JASMINE (*Jasminum officinale, J. odoratissimum*)
Flowers. One of the most expensive essential oils to buy. If you are fortunate enough to own some, you will cherish it for its incomparable fragrance. To capture some of the oil from your own plants you can infuse the jasmine flowers into oil for a soothing, sensual massage or bath oil. The dried flowers may be added to pillows to aid relaxation.

KAOLIN   A very fine earth clay powder with great absorption properties. Kaolin is used commercially for making porcelain, soap, paint and paper. Cosmetically it can be used as a base for masks and packs, particularly for oily/combination skins as it will absorb the grease from the skin.

LANOLIN, ANHYDROUS   Also known as 'wool fat'. This is a sticky yellow grease obtained by boiling the shorn wool of sheep. I stopped using lanolin for some time because of the many chemicals which were poured on the sheep's back. The new methods of treating sheep have resulted in purer lanolin but there will still be a pesticide residue in the wool fat if the sheep have grazed on pasture which has been treated with organophosphates, as these are deposited in the fat of both animals and humans and are cumulative. Much work is apparently being done on producing biodegradable pesticides which wouldn't present the risks to health that the present ones pose (unless you happen to be a ladybird, frog, praying mantis etc!!) I still can't come to terms with the use of pesticides and herbicides on such a scale.

The Food and Drug Authority has stated that the acceptable levels of pesticides in lanolin should be no more than five parts per million and this standard is one which is being used in Australia. I now feel that lanolin is probably a safer choice healthwise than petroleum jelly but I recommend nursing mothers try substituting cocoa butter and coconut oil in nipple creams instead of lanolin.

Lanolin is often sold as 'hydrous lanolin' which means that water has been beaten into the lanolin to make it more spreadable. All the recipes in this book contain 'anhydrous' (no water added) lanolin unless otherwise stated. Allergen.

LAVENDER (*Lavandula* sp.)   Leaves and flowers. One of the most useful cosmetic herbs. The leaves are almost as sweet smelling as the flowers, and are useful for adding bulk to mixtures for potpourris, sachets and pillows. Lavender blends well with rose and rosemary. Lavender oil is effective for soothing headaches if rubbed gently on the forehead, temples and base of the skull (don't get it in your eyes!). Added to massage oils to ease sore, aching muscles. Use the dried herb in facial steams, baths and astringents.

LECITHIN   Extracted mainly from soya beans and is of great value to the body both internally and externally. Granules are the best source of dietary lecithin as capsules contain too little lecithin to be effective unless taken in large quantities. It is also available as a thick syrupy liquid which may be used in hair conditioners and skin products.

Lecithin is found everywhere in the body and is utilised in the emulsifying of fats thus reducing the amount of cholesterol forming inside of arteries. It helps the body absorb and use vitamin B_6 and magnesium. Lecithin is reputed to be of assistance to those wishing to lose weight.

LEMON (*Citrus lemon*)   Whole fruit. Lemon oil is used in the perfume industry for its sharp, clean perfume. The skin and juice are acidic and may be added to baths, skin bleaches, facial steams or diluted as rinses for hair. If your elbows are scaly and discoloured, rest them in halved lemons to bleach and refine them. Mix juice with glycerine to soften chapped, rough hands. Add to lanolin to create an emulsion. Rub cut lemons on freckles and liver spots to fade them (follow with a moisture cream or lotion to counteract dryness).

LEMON BALM (*Melissa officinalis*)   Leaves. A perennial herb commonly known as 'lemon balm' or 'melissa'. This herb makes a delicious, refreshing, fever-reducing and soothing tea which helps to loosen and get rid of catarrh. An infusion may be used as an antiseptic cleansing wash for the face or in the bath, and in facial steams, hair rinses and shampoos. The essential oil is often used for allergies, asthma and menstrual problems.

LEMON GRASS (*Cymborpogon citratus*) Leaves. A tropical grass which grows well in Australia and other hot countries. Lemon grass is a good source of vitamin A. It normalises the action of the oil glands in the skin and is used in baths, steams and hair preparations, and as a wash for problem skins. Drunk as a tea it is pleasantly lemony and cooling.

LEMON VERBENA (*Lippia citriodora*) Leaves. When drunk as a tea, lemon verbena is a relaxant and a digestive. The lemon-scented leaves are used in facial steams, baths, potpourris, sachets and hair rinses. When dried, the leaves retain their perfume for years with no added fixative. I am still using lemon verbena which was dried six years ago!

LIME (*Citrus aurantifolia*) Whole fruit. Use in the same way as Lemon (see LEMON). Do not confuse with the Linden (see below).

LOOFAH (*Luffa cylindrica*) Years ago we planted loofahs against a long fence at our farm not knowing what to expect. They grew so large and heavy that we had to reinforce the fence. We picked thirty-eight loofahs from one plant alone! The loofah looks like a vegetable marrow and can be eaten but it doesn't have a very exciting flavour. When the loofah begins to get lighter in weight and the colour begins to turn from green to yellow it's ready for drying. Pick them off the vine and dump them in a bath, drum or similar container out of doors, cover with water and leave to rot, turning occasionally. The flesh will drop away leaving a fibrous skeleton. Wash the skeleton thoroughly but gently to get rid of any decayed vegetable matter and leave on a screen in a sunny airy place to dry. You now have wonderful, skin-stimulating loofahs to use in the bath and shower.

LOVAGE (*Levisticum officinalis*) Mainly root. Lovage is a perennial herb (to 1.5m/5ft) which looks and tastes much like celery. It has a deodorant effect as an infusion in the bath or as underarm splash.

MALLOW (*Malvaceae* sp.) Mainly root and leaves. There are many species of mallow, all of which are useful both internally and externally. The whole plant can be used but the root contains the greatest amount of mucilage. Be sure to prepare the root as soon as it's lifted—if you dry it first it becomes so tough that only an axe will chop it!

MARGARINE Margarine is an oil and water emulsion with chemicals added to give stability, flavour and colour. The oil phase may be animal or vegetable fat (sometimes a mixture of both). The fats are hydrogenated and chemicals are added in an unsuccessful attempt to emulate the smell and taste of butter. More chemicals are used to colour the product, artificial vitamins are added to 'enrich' the product and finally preservative is added to ensure a long shelf life! For more information on margarine and other foods I would urge you to read Consumer Beware! written by Beatrice Trum Hunter.

MARJORAM (*Origanum marjorana*) Leaves. Sweet marjoram is a perennial plant but gets quite woody so it's best to treat it as an annual. It is usually thought of as a culinary herb but in medieval days it was used as a strewing herb to improve and/or mask the smell of dwellings. The crushed herb may be held under the nose of a faint person (in the same way as smelling salts) and will revive them quickly. Marjoram adds a 'spicy' note to sweet bags, potpourris and herb pillows. A strong infusion in the bath or as a facial steam acts as a mild antiseptic and the vapours soothe the nervous system. This herb has a reputation for reducing sexual appetites but I can't make any person comment on that!

MAYONNAISE Mayonnaise contains eggs, vinegar or lemon juice, and oil—all of which are excellent to stimulate, nourish, moisturise and soften the skin and hair. If you don't want to make your own mayonnaise it's possible to buy soya mayonnaise (usually free from artificial additives) from health food shops. The addition of finely chopped herbs to the mayonnaise makes it even more luxurious for facials, packs, skin cream, or hair conditioner.

MELONS Flesh. Honeydew and rockmelon (cantaloupe) are suitable for dry skins; watermelon for oily or combination skins. The pulp may be used alone or mixed with any of the thickeners for a toning, cleansing mask (see Chapter Two).

MINTS (*Mentha* sp.)   Leaves. Mints are another of my 'top' cosmetic, cooking and medicinal herbs. The most important mints for cosmetic use are peppermint (*M. piperita*), spearmint (*M. viridis*) and eau de Cologne (*M. x piperita* 'Citrata').

The mints are aromatic, refreshing and restorative. Peppermint contains a large amount of menthol which leaves the skin feeling cool and stimulated. You will find many uses for mint in the recipes. Taken internally peppermint tea will relieve nervousness, headache, indigestion, stomach ache and nervous vomiting.

MOISTURISER   A liquid, lotion, cream or other agent which adds moisture to the skin or helps it to retain moisture.

MUCILAGE OR GEL   A jelly which can be used as an emollient base in many cosmetics, face masks and packs. Also used as a demulcent in medicinal preparations. For methods of making a mucilage or gel, see Chapter One.

MYRRH (*Commiphora myrrha*)   Resin. An exquisitely perfumed gum resin from the myrrh bush. The pale yellow resin is held in cavities in the bark from where it flows through fissures and hardens to walnut-sized, reddish-brown, brittle lumps. The sweet-smelling resin is used in incenses and perfumes where it acts as a fixative. It has astringent, antiseptic, anti-inflammatory and preservative properties. From this list you will see that myrrh is a most valuable ingredient in the making of mouthwashes, toothpowders, incense, ointments and creams. Include it in massage oils for its circulatory properties and perfume. See also the 'Directory of Essential Oils' in Chapter Six.

NETTLES (*Urtica dioica*)   Leaves. The ferocious stinging nettle becomes a 'pussy cat' after drying. It is one of the best hair herbs, particularly if drunk as a tea as well as used externally. It has the reputation of preventing hair loss and encouraging hair growth if used as an ingredient in shampoos or hair tonics. A strong infusion used in the bath or in facial steams will improve circulation and refine the skin.

NIGHT CREAM   A moisture cream which is usually heavier than that used during the daytime. The cream plumps the skin, softening lines and wrinkles, and also smooths the 'horny layer', making the skin texture softer.

OAK MOSS (*Evernia prunastri*)   A general term for various lichens which grow on oak trees. Oak moss is one of the oldest botanicals used by humans—it has been found in the tombs of Egyptian Pharaohs. When ground, it becomes the base for a body powder called 'chypre'. It is also used in soap making and as a fixative for potpourris. The scent of dried oak moss is sweet, musky and subtle.

OATS (*Avena sativa*)   If you have porridge left over from breakfast, save it until bathtime, fasten it in cheesecloth and dump it in your (or the baby's) bath. It will soften the water, soothe and smooth skin and get rid of itches. Use the bag as a washcloth—no need to use soap unless you are really grimy. There are many other ways to use oats: in masks; scrubs; soaps; and hand creams.

ORANGE (*Citrus* sp.)   Skin, flesh, juice, flowers, twigs, leaves. All parts of the orange are useful in making skin and hair care preparations. The oil in the peel is antiseptic and aromatic and may be used in moisture creams, toners, masks, bath mixtures, massage oils, shampoos and rinses. The oil is used in perfumery and for scenting creams and lotions. Orange-flower water may be used in cooking and in cosmetic making. As it doesn't keep fresh for very long it's best to use it in preparations which are made in small quantities and then refrigerated.

The flower of the orange tree is used in potpourris and massage oils. The flowers of the *Citrus bigardia* (bitter orange) are distilled to produce neroli oil. This oil is super-relaxing and is a 'base note' oil (see Chapter Six) which makes it very useful in perfume making. The leaves and twigs of the same tree are distilled to produce petitgrain oil. (The best oil is usually produced in France and North Africa.) It has a sharp, refreshing and relaxing scent used in perfumes.

ORRIS (*Iris florentina*)   Root. Orris is the violet-scented, dried, two-year-old rhizome of the

Florentine iris which has a bearded purple flower. The powdered root is used as a fixative in potpourris and perfumes. It is used in soap, body powders and toothpowders and pastes. Many people are allergic to it so test first. Allergen.

PAWPAW/PAPAYA (*Catica papaya*)   Flesh. This fruit contains enzymes which break down meat fibres (it can be used for tenderising steak) and acts as an exfoliant by removing the dead cells from the surface of the skin. I wouldn't suggest that you use this process too often but it's great when your skin feels and looks sallow and 'dead'. The pH of papaya is the same as skin. Allergen.

PARSLEY (*Petroselinum sativum*)   Leaves. This well-known herb is a diuretic and also contains lots of chlorophyll. The action of the diuretic is to flush the kidneys and the chlorophyll is a natural deodorant, so parsley eaten daily will give you a clear complexion and keep your breath sweet. It would be difficult to employ the chlorophyll as an external deodorant as the dye from parsley is a bright, most vivid green which would stain both clothes and armpits!

Parsley is rich in vitamin C. The infusion used as a skin wash cleanses oil from the skin. Its medicating properties are useful in creams, lotions and washes to help eczema and psoriasis.

PASSIONFLOWER (*Passiflora incarnata*)   Flower. This is the flower from the passionfruit vine. It makes a soothing and tranquillising infusion to drink or to use in a bath. The flower may be used when making massage oils, and sieved passionfruit pulp is a good additive to face masks.

PATCHOULI (*Pogostemon cablin, P. patchouli*)   Leaves. This is a very important perfume plant as the essential oil is a 'base note' and a fixative. Be very moderate with its use as it can overpower. The perfume is stimulating and quite intense—it brings back memories of my visits to India where the oil is used extensively as a perfume and the leaves laid between cloth to protect it from insects.

PEACH (*Prunus persica*)   Fruit, leaves. The flesh, oil and the aromatic leaves may be used. The mashed flesh is moisturising and softening to dry, rough skin. The leaves, which are emollient, may be chopped, made into an infusion and used in masks and baths. Peach kernel oil (see FIXED OILS) is fine, delicate and expensive so I reserve it for the most luxurious products.

PEAR (*Pyrus communis*)   Fruit. The slight grittiness and mild acidity of mashed pear flesh makes it an ideal addition to facial masks. The flesh is soothing and cooling to sun or windburnt skin.

PECTIN   A mildly acidic extract from the inner pulp of citrus rind and from crushed apple pulp. Pectin makes an excellent gel which has the correct pH for skin. See Chapter One.

PENNYROYAL (*Mentha pulegium*)   Leaves. A member of the mint family which can become very invasive if not kept in check. Pennyroyal used externally is a good flea and mosquito repellent. The Latin name *pulegium* means flea—so named for its reputation for repelling fleas when used externally on animals and their bedding. It may be used in the bath for its perfume, skin soothing, deodorant properties. *Caution: Pennyroyal is quite a powerful abortifacient and must never be used during pregnancy. Allergen.*

PETROLEUM JELLY   If you feel at all dubious about using lanolin in your ointments (see LANOLIN) you can use petroleum jelly as a substitute. It will provide softness to counteract the hardness of beeswax but it doesn't add any goodness to the preparation in the way that lanolin does and may contain many undesirable chemicals.

pH   A number used to express degrees of acidity or alkalinity. Litmus paper is used to establish whether a liquid is acid or alkaline. Blue litmus turns red (indicating an acid if the pH is below 7.0, stays blue (indicating an alkaline) if the pH is above 7.0. The average pH of skin is 5.5 and should be aimed at in home-made preparations.

PHENOXITOL   See PRESERVATIVES.

PHOTOSENSITIVITY   A condition where the skin becomes oversensitive to light after the application of certain substances. The skin may develop rashes, swellings, redness or hyperpigmentation.

PINE (*Pinus* sp.)   Needles, oil. The clean, fresh, forest smell of pine makes it an ideal herb for incenses cones, toilet and room refreshers, aftershave lotions and skin toners, massage oils for tired muscles, and aromatic pillows. Pineapple (*Ananas comosus*)   Flesh. Like the pawpaw (papaya), pineapple contains enzymes which can tenderise meat—this makes it useful as an exfoliant. I become very aware of the enzymes when I try to eat raw pineapples—I love the flavour but my lips become sore very quickly. The enzyme is inactivated by heat and I can eat canned pineapple with no ill effects. Mild allergen.

PLANTAIN (*Plantago major, P. lanceolata*)   Whole herb. A perennial herb which is considered a bit of a pest by those who don't know its value. The astringent action of the crushed leaf takes the pain out of ant and bee stings, and the same action makes this a very useful herb when made into lotions and face masks for oily or inflamed skin. Mild allergen.

POTATO (*Solanum tuberosum*)   Mashed potato makes a healing treatment for rough chapped hands. Grated raw potato can be used as a poultice to get rid of bruising, and if soaked in a glass of water overnight and drunk in the morning will de-acidify the system.

POULTICE   A pulped, heated mass of herbs, vegetables or other agents usually enclosed in cloth and applied to the skin to relieve congestion or to draw pus or foreign bodies from a wound.

PRESERVATIVES   I recently spoke at length to a very reputable chemist who works for a large, well-known pharmaceutical company. The subject of the conversation was preservatives. The recommendations he made to me (for inclusion in this book) were based on the low allergenic properties and low toxicity of certain preservatives.

Without the addition of preservatives, most home-made preparations which contain moist ingredients will last for only a few days, even with refrigeration. In order to achieve a reasonable shelf life for your products, it is necessary to use some form of preservative which either kills or inhibits the growth of bacteria.

One of the prime causes of deterioration of creams and lotions is the use of fingers to take cream out of a jar. Even after washing, our skin is inhabited by millions of microscopic creatures which we transfer to the contents of the jar every time we stick our fingers in. The use of a 'pop stick' to take creams and ointments out of containers will lengthen the life of the contents quite dramatically.

Many preservatives such as glycerine, tincture of benzoin, citric acid and benzoic acid are wholly natural but have as many drawbacks as synthetically produced preservatives. Benzoic acid, for instance, is an allergen to many people and can cause symptoms which range from mild itching to the outbreak of a severe rash. To be an effective preservative, 20% glycerine would be needed in a recipe but this amount would have the effect of drawing moisture from your skin rather than the desired effect of drawing water into your skin from the atmosphere.

The decisions you have to make are based on several factors:

(a) The time you have available to make the preparations. If time is of no consequence and you can make fresh batches every few days, refrigeration is all that is required.

(b) Are the preparations for your own use or to give as gifts? If the latter applies, a preservative will be needed unless the recipient is aware that the lotion etc. has a short life.

(c) If distilled/purified water is used instead of juices or herb waters, the bacterial action is lessened.

(d) Water-in-oil preparations (such as healing ointments) have a much longer life than oil-in-water emulsions as oil itself acts as a preservative. Oil can oxidise and become rancid but some oils (semi-drying and drying) resist oxidisation better than others. These oils however, have the disadvantage of becoming quite sticky after a long period of storing. I was recently shown an almost empty jar of Green Healer which I made about ten years ago—it was tacky and sticky but was still doing a good job of healing cuts and sores.

(e) A bottle of lotion which is unpreserved and which has developed bacterial action presents far more of a risk than a similar bottle which has had a chemical preservative added. You wouldn't consider eating food which had gone bad as you know that it would make you ill—cosmetics which have gone bad will make your skin ill and spotty.

The two chemical preservatives which I have used successfully and with no reported ill effects are chlorocresol and phenoxitol. They are not as strong as many used by commercial cosmetic manufacturers but were recommended to me by two very reputable pharmaceutical chemists, and a dermatologist who uses them in ointments and creams for healing skin problems. These two preservatives are both water-miscible and are added to the water phase in products.

Caution: The recommended proportions need to be adhered to very precisely and must never be exceeded: phenoxitol is used at a concentration of 1% (that is 1g to every 99g (3^1/$_3$oz) of other ingredients); chlorocresol is used at a concentration of 0.1% (that is ^{1}/$_{10}$th of a gram (1mg) to 99.9g (3^1/$_3$oz) of other ingredients).

Unless you are making a large quantity it becomes obvious that phenoxitol is the easier to use, as without very fine laboratory scales it would be impossible to weigh the minute amount of chlorocresol required. A compromise between using no preservative or a chemical preservative would be to add 10% glycerine combined with 4% tincture of benzoin to an appropriate preparation. I can't tell you for how long the mixture would be preserved as this would depend on many factors: method of storage, other ingredients, sterility of contents and containers.

QUINCE (*Pyrus cydonia, Cydonia oblonga*)   The seeds of the quince are used to make a mucilage or gel. It is soothing and emollient and may be used as a thickener, toner or aftershave lotion. For instructions on making the gel see Chapter One.

ROCKROSE (*Cistus ladanifer*)   Leaf. A large shrub up to 2m (6^1/$_2$ft) with long, dark green sticky leaves and large, thin petalled white flowers which have a maroon 'splodge' at the base of the petals. The dried leaves make a good fixative in potpourris.

ROSE (*Rosa* sp.)   Petals. The main varieties from which rose oil is extracted are: *Rosa gallica* (French rose), *R. damascena* (damask rose), *R. centifolia*

(cabbage rose). It takes about thirty roses to get one drop of oil which is why the oil is so expensive. There are many synthetics on the market so if you find an inexpensive rose oil the chances are that it's not the real thing. The oil is used in expensive cosmetics and perfumery, and also to make rose-water (see later). An infusion from rose petals is gently astringent, soothing and hydrating.

ROSEMARY (*Rosmarinus officinalis*)   Leaves. One of the best known and loved herbs. Rosemary has dark green, spiky leaves and blue flowers. When you strip the leaves from the stem your fingers become sticky from the aromatic resinous oil which is freely released from the plant. Rosemary is a good addition to baths and facial steams (particularly if you are suffering from 'brain fag'), shampoos and rinses, perfumes, toilet and room fresheners, disinfectants and insecticides.

ROSE-WATER   A scented water made from rose petals or rose oil. Triple rose-water (which may be bought from pharmacies) is prepared by distillation of fresh blooms of Rosa damascena. To use, add one part rose-water to two parts purified water. The resulting rose-water can be used in cleansing creams, toners, moisture lotions and as a toilet water.

RUBEFACIENT   An agent which reddens the skin by bringing an increased blood supply to the area. Chilli has this property.

SAGE (*Salvia officinalis*)   Leaves. Well-known perennial herb. Both the red sage and common garden sage may be used for their disinfectant, soothing and astringent properties. A chewed leaf eases and often cures mouth ulcers. Infusions are used in shampoos and rinses for dark hair and facial rinses for pimply skin. An infusion in the bath helps to check excessive perspiration.

ST JOHN'S WORT (*Hypericum perforatum*)   Leaves, flowers. A perennial herb which has transparent spots on the leaves; these are sacs which carry the volatile oil. The five-petalled flowers are yellow and have black glands spotting the edges. The glands contain a dark red oil. The extracted oil is healing and regenerative—it's suitable for massage oils, creams and lotions for dry, rough skin.

SANDALWOOD (*Santalum album*)   Dried wood. Sandalwood oil is distilled from the heart wood of trees that are twenty to thirty years old. The wood only develops its distinctive perfume when it is dried. The oil is used for its perfume and disinfectant/antiseptic properties in soaps, incense, air fresheners and perfumes, and as a fixative in potpourris, sweet bags and perfumes.

SLIPPERY ELM POWDER   The dried and ground inner bark of the North American tree *Ulmus fulva*. This species of tree is becoming endangered due to commercial overfarming so I restrict its use in my household to internal, medicinal use when there is a case of vomiting or diarrhoea and 'sore tummy'.

SOAPWORT (*Saponaria officinalis*)   The root and to a lesser degree the twigs and leaves contain a saponin which is useful when made into a decoction and included in shampoos. The lather isn't abundant but the cleansing effect is thorough and gentle. The decoction has been used to restore and clean delicate silks and tapestries.

SODIUM SESQUICARBONATE   A mixture of washing soda (sodium carbonate) and bicarbonate of soda (sodium bicarbonate) which is used in bath preparations as a water softener.

SOUTHERNWOOD (*Artemisia abrotanum*)   Leaves. A pungently scented perennial herb with a shrublike growth. The leaves are thin and needle-like. Use an infusion for an invigorating, disinfectant bath which stimulates the circulation; use in a wash for pimply skin and a rinse for hair (said to stimulate growth); use in air freshener and insect repellent mixtures.

STORAX (STYRAX) (*Liquidambar orientalis*)   A balsam formed in damaged bark of the tree. The bark is collected, peeled and boiled to obtain raw storax which is then purified to a syrupy, delicately perfumed substance. Storax is used in perfumes as a fixative and in soaps, creams and lotions for the scent. Unfortunately it's becoming increasingly difficult to buy.

STRAWBERRY (*Frageria* sp.)   Leaves, fruit. The leaves of this well-known plant are used as astringent infusions in baths and as facial washes for oily skin. The mashed fruit is used as a mask for oily, blemished skin. The fruit is also rubbed on teeth to whiten them and remove stains.

STYPTIC   As astringent agent which contracts tissue and is often used to stop bleeding.

TALCUM POWDER   A mixture of various chalks which are milled until very fine. It's most important to use only pharmaceutical standard, sterilised talcum—earthborne bacteria such as tetanus may be contained in unsterilised chalk. These bacteria could cause illness and in the case of small babies, death. Sterilise dubious talcum in a 150°C (300°F) oven for one hour, stirring often.

TARTARIC ACID   An acid found in many fruits, particularly grapes. Tartaric acid is produced commercially from the lees of winemaking. It is used in fizzy drinks and bath salts.

TEA BAGS   Tea contains tannin which is an astringent, so the good old tea bag is useful for soothing the pain of sunburn and if laid on the eyes will reduce under-eye puffiness and relieve eye strain. To avoid staining your skin you should smear a little oil under the eyes first.

THYME (*Thymus* sp.)   Leaves. 'An annual herb with many cosmetic, medicinal and household uses. Thyme is antiseptic, aromatic, disinfectant, and diaphoretic. Use it in deodorants, mouthwashes, bath mixtures, shampoos and hair rinses, aftershaves, facial steams and masks.

THYMOL   An aromatic crystalline phenol extracted from thyme (*Thymus vulgaris*). Thymol is powerfully antibacterial and antiseptic.

TINCTURE   A method of preserving the properties of herbs by extraction into an alcoholic solution. For method of making, see Chapter One.

TOMATO (*Lycopersicon esculentum*)   Tomatoes are acidic which makes them good for controlling oil on greasy skins. Use in masks to refine coarse skin.

TONIC   A stimulant, usually liquid, which restores vigour and health to a depleted system.

TRAGACANTH (*Astralagus gummifer*) A gum obtained from a small thorny shrub. When dried and powdered, the gum is pale yellow to beige. Tragacanth is very expensive but very little is needed as it's such a powerful thickening agent. See Chapter One. Mild allergen.

TRIETHANOLAMINE A substance formed from ammonia and alcohol which is used in conjunction with stearic acid and other ingredients to make vanishing creams. See EMULSIFYING WAX.

UNGUENT Another word for ointment.

VASELINE See PETROLEUM JELLY.

VINEGAR The word 'vinegar' is derived from the French vin aigre which means sour wine. Cider vinegar is made from apples, and wine vinegars from grapes; these are the two most suitable for cosmetic use. Malt and other vinegars are too harsh for use on skin.

VIOLET (*Viola odorata*) Flowers, leaves. Violets are hardy perennials. Both leaves and flowers are soothing, mildly astringent and are rich in vitamins A and C, making them very suitable for use in creams, lotions and toners for all skins. The infusion is gentle enough to use on a baby's skin. Flowers are lovely in potpourris, pillows and sachets.

WASHING SODA (SODIUM CARBONATE) A mixture of soda ash and sodium carbonate available as powder or crystals used for softening water. Washing soda solution is very alkaline and has the potential to burn or severely irritate skin and mucous membranes. It may be mixed with bicarbonate of soda to create sodium sesquicarbonate, a less alkaline mixture. When using washing soda, wear gloves and avoid inhaling the powder.

WATER A good medium for the growth of bacteria. As water is often the largest proportion of any of the recipes in this book, it's necessary to use purified or distilled water to ensure that the preparations last as long as possible.

A piece of cotton wool squeezed out in cold water and patted on the face will 'set' make-up and help it to last longer. Drinking six to eight glasses of water daily will keep your system flushed out and help to keep your skin and eyes clear. In winter, when heaters are drying the air and your skin, a bowl of water in the room will humidify the air and your skin will thank you for it.

WATERMELON (*Citrullus vulgaris*) Flesh. This delicious, thirst-quenching fruit has a pH very close to that of skin. It's also very high in betacarotene. Use the juice as a facial wash and the mashed fruit as a mask.

WILLOW, WHITE (*Salix alba*) Bark. The dried bark is very astringent. A decoction makes an excellent wash for eczema, psoriasis, pimples and oily skin. Use also in aftershaves and deodorants.

Caution: Willow contains salicylates which are common allergens.

WITCH HAZEL (*Hamamelis virginiana*) Bark, leaves and distilled witch hazel extract. In this book you will find many uses for distilled witch hazel extract, particularly for toners and astringents. The leaves and bark of this shrub are very astringent, styptic and cleansing. An infusion reduces skin inflammation, the pain of stings, dandruff, bruises and swellings. Because of its astringency it is a most useful toner for oily skin and is a reasonably good deodorant for both underarm and vaginal areas. Distilled witch hazel extract is readily available from pharmacies.

YARROW (*Achillea millefolium*) Leaves. A biennial herb which has a healing and astringent action. Useful for facials, douches, shampoos and mouthwashes (particularly if there is inflammation present). If mixed with peppermint leaves and elderflowers and drunk as a tea it is an excellent cold and flu cure. Added to the bath it helps to heal eczema.

ZINC OXIDE A soft, heavy, white powder which when added to creams forms a soothing, mildly astringent protective barrier. Very suitable for application to babies' bottoms.

BOOK LIST

AROMATHERAPY AND FRAGRANCES

Aromatherapy, Nerys Purchon (Hodder & Stoughton, 1994).

Aromatherapy, Robert Tisserand (Granada, 1977).

The Illustrated Herbal, Nicholas Culpeper (Harvey Sales, 1981).

Herbs and Aromatherapy, Joannah Metcalf (Webb & Bower, 1989).

The Fragrant Pharmacy, Valerie Ann Worwood (Bantam Books, 1991).

The Directory of Essential Oils, Wanda Sellar (C.W. Daniel Co. Ltd, 1992)

The Encyclopaedia of Essential Oils, Julia Lawless (Element Books Limited, 1992)

COSMETICS

Cosmetic & Fragrance Book, Elizabeth Franke (Simon & Schuster, 1988).

Cosmetics and How to Make Them, Robert Bushby (Pitman, 1947).

Formulation & Function of Cosmetics, Joseph Stefan Jellinek (Wiley Interscience, 1970).

Herbal Delights, Mrs Carl F. Leyel (Faber, 1987).

Herbal Body Book, Jeanne Rose (Grosset & Dunlap, 1976).

Making Your Own Cosmetics, James Sholto Douglas (Pelham Books, 1979).

Natural Beauty, Lorna Horrocks (Angus & Robertson, 1980).

Natural Beauty Book, Clare Maxwell-Hudson (MacDonald, 1976).

New Unguent Bases and Lotions, Hoffman (Chemical Publishing, 1957).

Super Hair, Zizmor & John Forman (Berkley, 1978).

Super Skin, Nelson Lee Novick (Clarkson N. Potter, 1988).

FOOD

Dictionary of Nutritional Health, Adrienne Mayes (Lothian, 1986).

Food: What's In It, Catherine Saxelby (Reed Books, 1989).

Consumer Beware!, Beatrice Trum Hunter (Simon & Schuster, 1971).

Nutrition for Life, Catherine Saxelby (Reed Books, 1986).

Additive Code Breaker, Maurice Hanssen (Lothian, 1991).

Complete Book of Food & Nutrition, Rosemary Stanton (Simon & Schuster, 1989).

Eating for Life, Rosemary Stanton (Murdoch Books, 1992).

Diet for a Small Planet, Frances Moore Lappe (Ballantyne, 1972).

Fat is a Feminist Issue, Susie Orbach (Hamlyn, 1978).

F-Plan Diet, Audrey Eyton (Penguin, 1982).

F+, Audrey Eyton (Penguin, 1984).

Health on your Plate, Janette Pleshette (Arrow Books, 1983).

The Book of Tofu, W. Shurtleff & A. Aoyagi (Ballantyne, 1979).

The Food Pharmacy, Jean Carper (Simon & Schuster, 1988).

The 8-week Cholesterol Cure, Robert E. Kowalski (Bantam Schwartz, 1987).

Thinning from the Inside Out, Elizabeth Lay (Bantam Books, 1986).

The 3D Slimming Diet, Michael Spira (Corgi, 1984).

GENERAL

Herbcraft, Nerys Purchon (Hodder & Stoughton, 1995).

Martindale Pharmacopoeia (Pharmaceutical Press, 1982).

Meditation

The Orange Book, Bhagwan Shree Rajneesh (Rajneesh Foundation International, 1981).

Complete Meditation, Steve Kravette (Para Research, 1982).

GUIDE TO MEASURES

As the enjoyment of good home-made food and the love of cooking spreads throughout the world, it's important to have easy-to-follow conversion of measures in our recipes. In some countries they use metric measures, in others imperial measures, and many cooks like to use handy cup and spoon measures. In Australia, we use metric measures and cup and spoon measures approved by the Standards Association of Australia.

➤ The metric measuring cup holds 250ml
➤ The metric measuring tablespoon holds 20ml
➤ The metric measuring teaspoon holds 5ml

The conversions given in the recipes in this book are approximate. Any differences should not make any noticeable difference to these recipes. We use 60g (2oz) eggs in our recipes.

Dry Measures		Liquid Measures		Helpful Measures	
METRIC	IMPERIAL	METRIC	IMPERIAL	METRIC	IMPERIAL
15g	½oz	30ml	1 fluid oz	3mm	⅛in
30g	1oz	60ml	2 fluid oz	6mm	¼in
60g	2oz	100ml	3 fluid oz	1cm	½in
90g	3oz	125ml	4 fluid oz	2cm	¾in
100g	3½oz	150ml	5 fluid oz	2.5cm	1in
125g	4oz (¼lb)		(¼ pint/1 gill)	5cm	2in
155g	5oz	185ml	6 fluid oz	6cm	2½in
185g	6oz	250ml	8 fluid oz	8cm	3in
200g	6½oz	300ml	10 fluid oz	10cm	4in
220g	7oz		(½ pint)	13cm	5in
250g	8oz (½lb)	500ml	16 fluid oz	15cm	6in
280g	9oz	750ml	24 fluid oz	18cm	7in
315g	10oz	1000ml (1 litre)	32 fluid oz	20cm	8in
345g	11oz		(1¾ pints)	23cm	9in
375g	12oz (¾lb)			25cm	10in
410g	13oz			28cm	11in
440g	14oz			30cm	12in (1ft)
470g	15oz				
500g	16oz (1lb)				
750g	24oz (1½lb)				
1kg	32oz (2lb)				

Oven Temperatures

These oven temperatures are only a guide. Always check the manufacturer's manual.

	C (CELSIUS)	F (FAHRENHEIT)	GAS MARK
Very slow	120	250	1
Slow	150	300	2
Moderately slow	160	325	3
Moderate	180	350	4
Moderately hot	190	375	5
Hot	200	400	6
Very hot	230	450	7

INDEX